Complementary Medicine:

a practical guide

Complementary Medicine:
a practical guide

Tanvir Jamil BSc, BM, MRCGP
General Practitioner, Buckinghamshire, UK

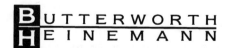

Butterworth-Heinemann
Linacre House, Jordan Hill, Oxford OX2 8DP
A division of Reed Educational and Professional Publishing Ltd

℞ A member of the Reed Elsevier plc group

OXFORD   BOSTON   JOHANNESBURG
MELBOURNE   NEW DELHI   SINGAPORE

First published 1997

© Reed Educational and Professional Publishing Ltd 1997

British Library Cataloguing in Publication Data
A catalogue record for this book is available from the British Library

Library of Congress Cataloguing in Publication Data
A catalogue record for this book is available from the Library of Congress

ISBN 0 7506 2881 2

Typeset by BC Typesetting, Bristol BS18 1NZ
Printed and bound in Great Britain by Biddles Ltd, Guildford and King's Lynn

For
Hasham and Sumira

Contents

Part Two Common conditions and their treatment

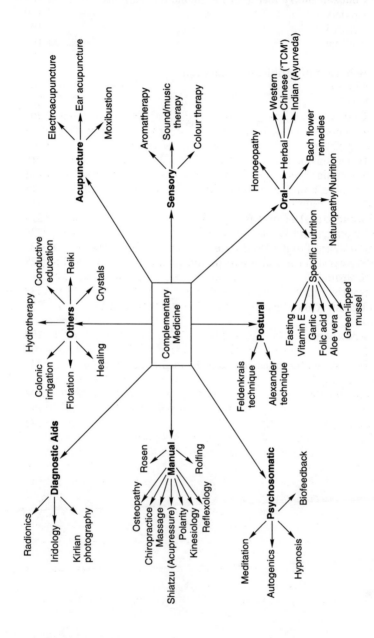

Figure A Complementary medicine

Preface

Welcome to this book. Whether you work in orthodox medicine (doctor, medical student, nurse, physiotherapist, etc.) or in complementary therapy, or are a potential patient, this book has been designed to help you find out more about specific complementary therapies: what they are, how they work, what they treat, what they cannot treat, where to find a practitioner and where to train.

More doctors are now being asked about complementary medicine by an increasingly aware public. Acupuncture and osteopathy are well known, but how do you go about helping patients whose minds are set on rolfing, sound therapy or the Alexander technique? I hope this book will assist all those general practitioners who have come across this problem and would like to find out more. You may even decide to incorporate some of these therapies into your own practice.

If you are not medically qualified, please do not be put off by the fact that the book is suitable for 'medics'. I have tried to write clearly and without the use of jargon. Where jargon is used I have explained it in parenthesis or in the glossary. If you are interested in complementary therapy generally or wish to follow a career in a therapy, or have a problem you think may be helped, this book will point you in the right direction. I have also included advice on self-help measures which may give you greater insight into the therapy and hopefully benefit your health at the same time.

I have tried to keep the history and philosophy behind each therapy as brief as possible. I have used bullet points and brief notes liberally and hope this has resulted in an interesting book that can be used for quick reference.

Every effort has been made to check each organization's address and telephone number. If details change please let me know by way of Butterworth-Heinemann.

This book contains details of over 70 therapies. A few such as yoga have not been included, primarily because these are self-help methods ideal for the healthy. Some of the more obscure therapies such as urine therapy and pearl therapy have also been excluded; I felt that these were too marginal to be included in this book.

Orthodox medicine can learn a great deal from the positive attitudes of complementary therapy towards health, well-being, healing and holistic treatment. Unfortunately there is still some mistrust between these two spheres of medicine. Many doctors are unhappy with referring patients to therapists owing to a lack of supporting evidence. Perhaps our attitude should be this: if the patient benefits it really does not matter how or why the therapy works, the patient's quality of life is paramount.

M. T. J.
June 1997

Acknowledgements

I should like to thank my wife, Sumira, for help with researching this book and reading the manuscript. Her good humour, patience and excellent cooking have sustained me through the marathon that books inevitably become.

Thanks also to my father Muhammad Jamil and my mother Anwar Jamil for pushing me when I needed it and educating me in life.

My sisters Ghazala and Shehla, and my brother Naveed need a special mention. Thanks for all your encouragement over the years.

I am grateful to my friend and colleague Bev Daily and Mary Seager of Butterworth-Heinemann for their advice and support in the writing of this book.

M.T.J.

Part One
Complementary therapies

An overview of complementary medicine

Nomenclature

'Alternative' medicine has been defined as health care that lies for the most part outside the mainstream of orthodox medicine. With an increasing number of alternatives to choose from and the acceptance of some into modern medicine there have been several moves away from the term 'alternative':

- 'Complementary' – the most widely used term.
- 'Complementary' and 'non-conventional'. The former term indicates self-contained medical systems with their own ideas on aetiology (cause of disease) and diagnosis, e.g. homoeopathy, acupuncture, Chinese herbal medicine and ayurveda. The latter term indicates other practices such as reflexology, healing, hypnosis, etc.
- A detailed classification has been suggested by Wardwell in the USA. Alternative health professions would be subdivided into 'ancillary' (e.g. osteopathy, acupuncture, homoeopathy), 'limited' (e.g. herbal medicine, hypnosis), 'marginal' (e.g. reflexology, Alexander technique) and 'quasi' (e.g. healing, iridology).

Facts, figures and trends

Patient demand for complementary medicine grew throughout the 1980s. By the end of the decade more doctors were becoming interested too.

- Ten per cent of the British public visit a complementary therapist.
- In the UK the most prevalent therapies are manipulation (used by 36% of the population), herbalism (24%), homoeopathy (16%) and acupuncture (16%).

- More than two-thirds of general practitioners (GPs) refer or direct patients to complementary practitioners. Most referrals are, however, patient-initiated.

In 1993 the National Health Service in the UK spent £1 million on complementary medicine either in GP surgeries or directly in hospitals. Some of the more unusual therapies paid for include healing and transcendental meditation. A large number of NHS referrals go to the Royal London Homoeopathic Hospital or the Glasgow Homoeopathic Hospital. With the introduction of fund-holding some GPs have privately employed complementary practitioners (e.g. osteopaths) in their surgeries.

- Aromatherapy, reflexology and massage are available in 90% of palliative care settings (e.g. cancer and AIDS wards) in the UK.
- In the South West Thames area 1 in 5 GPs and 1 in 8 hospital consultants practise a complementary therapy.
- In Canada 65% of GPs perceived a demand for complementary medicine from their patients.
- During 1990 complementary medicine was used by 1 in 3 Americans and 1 in 4 saw a conventional doctor also.

The role of the nurse is slowly shifting from caregiver to healer. General practitioners are employing more 'nurse practitioners' to deal with uncomplicated medical problems. Hospital nurses and midwives are being encouraged to incorporate complementary therapies into their skill mix, such as aromatherapy, massage, yoga, guided imagery, therapeutic touch, reflexology and music therapy.

Dangers of complementary therapy

Lack of government regulation means that anyone can take a weekend course and then set up as a complementary therapist and start seeing patients. Inexperienced practitioners may treat a serious underlying illness and not refer the patient back to a medically qualified doctor. The rapid rise in herbal medicine, especially the use of Chinese herbal cures, has led to a large number of toxic events. Complementary therapies also have the disadvantage of being generally more expensive than conventional treatment.

Although an increasing amount of research is being carried out into the main complementary therapies there are still many practices based purely on ancient beliefs without any scientific foundation.

Why do people see complementary therapists?

- Recommendation from GP, friend, advertisement, radio, magazine, etc.
- Lack of time in conventional medical consultations to provide comfort, counselling and support. The average complementary therapist offers a 1-hour initial consultation then 15–45 minutes for follow-up visits.
- A wish to be cured 'holistically', not just by removal of symptoms.
- A wish for a firm diagnostic label for each illness.
- An attraction to remedies based on ancient beliefs that retain an essential degree of mystery.
- A wish for 'natural' therapies.
- Therapists often prescribe 'nice' rather than 'nasty' treatments.
- Favourable media coverage.
- Education and awareness: patients who use therapies are often middle-aged women from social classes 1 and 2. Children seeing complementary practitioners differ significantly from those who only use conventional medicine in that their parents are better educated and also use similar therapies.
- Patients consult practitioners for mild to moderate long-term, painful, functional and stress-related conditions. Patients with chronic incurable disease, e.g. diabetes, for which orthodox medicinal treatment is somewhat unsatisfactory, also seek complementary therapy.
- Many complementary therapies will not cure but can have a positive effect on quality of life.

Guidelines for patients

See your GP for advice and to rule out any serious causes of illness. This is particularly important if you are under medical treatment already. The GP may recommend a complementary therapist. If not, try to obtain one by recommendation or by telephoning the professional organizations listed in this book for a list of practitioners in your local area.

Many therapists are happy to talk over the telephone or at their clinic before instigating treatment. Ask about experience in treating your condition, length of course, fees and side-effects. Ask if the therapist will be communicating with your GP. Before treatment, check credentials, attitudes to health, standards at the clinic and quality of staff.

Be realistic in your expectations – do not expect a miracle cure. Be prepared to take responsibility for your own health. This is true for *all* types of medical care. Many complementary practitioners will give advice and exercises that must be followed at home regularly.

Pay for one session only at first and try it. If it is unsuitable, stop and try something else.

The vast majority of therapists are happy to work with patients on conventional medication. In the unlikely event of a therapist asking you to stop all your medication, ignore this advice and see your GP. Do not use more than two complementary therapies simultaneously. Many therapies complement each other, e.g. acupuncture and manipulation; others can have unfavourable interactions, e.g. homoeopathy and aromatherapy. Check with the practitioners involved.

If there is no benefit after a recommended course of treatment – stop. Either try something else or see your GP.

Many orthodox doctors are still wary of complementary therapies primarily because of a lack of supporting evidence. As long you have checked with your doctor that your condition is not serious, go ahead and see a therapist as outlined above. *If* you can afford it, *if* it suits you *and* you feel better it does not really matter *how* it works.

2

Acupuncture

Background

Acupuncture probably dates back 5000 years and the earliest known text on the subject is the Yellow Emperor's classic of internal medicine (*Nei Jing*) which was written between 475 and 221 BC. It is still available from bookshops today.

The Chinese may have stumbled on the idea when soldiers wounded by arrows were sometimes cured of acute or chronic ailments in parts of the body distant from the wound. In time such arrow wounds were imitated with needles made from bamboo, stone and bone to help cure the sick. The Chinese realized that the size of the wound was not important, the crucial factor was its position in the body. From these early days of trial and error the complex art of traditional acupuncture developed. The relationships between needling and cure were established and passed on from generation to generation.

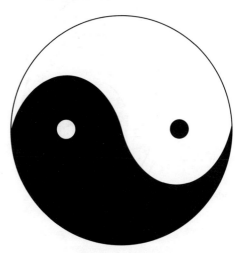

Figure 2.1 Yin and yang

A philosophy evolved to explain how and why acupuncture worked. A circulation of energy (*chi*) was described within the body and consisted of deep and superficial components (*yin* and *yang*) which met at the surface of the body in strategic areas – acupuncture points. An imbalance of *chi* was thought to cause disease. Needling of strategically chosen acupuncture points was believed to realign *yin* and *yang* and in turn *chi*. Figure 2.1 illustrates the symbol for *yin* and *yang*, indicating the perfect balance and constant interaction of energies in healthy existence.

Acupuncture was introduced into Europe in the seventeenth century, but knowledge of the art was very patchy until 1970 when President Nixon's visit to China opened the floodgates to the West. Europe has, however, made one significant contribution to acupuncture. In the 1950s the Frenchman Nogier mapped out a series of points for ear acupuncture (auricular therapy). The work by Nogier was highly respected and his teachings have now been incorporated into Chinese acupuncture.

Pulse and tongue diagnosis are offshoots of acupuncture that arose from ancient cultural teachings to maintain modesty. Thus the practitioner was only presented with the forearms, the lower legs and the tongue (Figure 2.2) with which to make a diagnosis. He would examine the radial pulses, look for changes on the surface of the tongue and formulate his diagnosis.

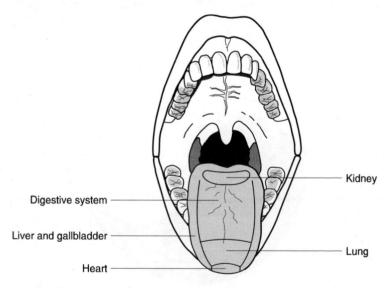

Figure 2.2 Tongue diagnosis

Chinese physiology also categorized disease into 'cold' and 'damp' and thus a method of 'warming' was used whereby moxa wool (made from the dried leaves of the common mugwort, *Artemisia vulgaris*) was burnt on the end of a needle.

The acupuncture practised today postulates the existence of a series of 14 meridians and over 2000 acupuncture points. Meridians are imaginary lines joining a series of acupuncture points. Each has a name which is usually taken from one of the internal organs. For example, the 'colon' meridian starts at the tip of the index finger, runs up the arm and over the shoulder to end at the side of the nose. The other meridians similarly criss-cross the body. Such meridian and acupuncture charts are widely available (Figure 2.3) illustrating the human body and, for veterinary practitioners, cats, dogs and elephants.

Research

Double-blind controlled studies, where the clinician is ignorant of the treatment allocation, cannot be easily applied or maintained in acupuncture. Definition of an appropriate control group is also difficult. Controls used in various trials have included:

● An alternative treatment group: for example, comparison with patients receiving transcutaneous electrical nerve stimulation (TENS).
● Acupuncture at non-classical sites or 'sham' acupuncture, i.e. needle insertion away from precise acupuncture points.

The problem is, however, that TENS and sham acupuncture have their own definite therapeutic benefits. Therefore more recent trials have tended to use other controls:

● Mock TENS, i.e. the machine is attached but not switched on.
● Minimal acupuncture: sham acupuncture involving minimal surface stimulation. This procedure minimizes the specific effects of needling while maintaining the psychological impact.
● A 'no treatment' or waiting-list group.

In spite of the methodological problems there have been many excellent studies on acupuncture in the last 20 years which clearly indicate its effectiveness and validity. In summary, the trials have shown:

● Acupuncture analgesia is reproducible in laboratory conditions.
● Levels of endorphins are raised after acupuncture treatment.

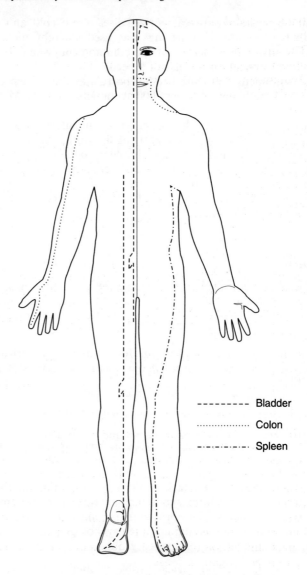

Figure 2.3 Acupuncture meridians

- Immunoglobulin levels in rheumatoid patients can be affected by acupuncture treatment.
- The effects of acupuncture may be reversed by naloxone – an opioid antagonist that inhibits the action of endorphins.
- Acupuncture can work in animals.
- Trials with sham acupuncture indicate that the true technique reduces pain better.

Other studies have shown the beneficial effects of acupuncture on pain relief (back pain, migraines, arthritis, postoperative pain, renal colic and menstrual pain), nausea and vomiting, and on asthma and substance abuse. Many general practitioners and specialists feel that acupuncture has a future in orthodox medicine. Protocols for research are being developed, good quality research is in progress and leading journals are publishing more papers.

Mechanism of action

The abstract concepts of *chi*, *yin* and *yang* and much of the philosophical theory of traditional acupuncture is looked upon with some scepticism by modern medical practitioners. However, scientific research (see above) has helped to concentrate thinking on several possible mechanisms:

- Endorphins and enkephalins (the body's natural opioid or narcotic-like hormones) are released which affect the central nervous system, blocking pain and altering control of bodily organs.
- 'Closing the gate': the 'gate' theory of pain suggests pain impulses have to travel through a gate in the nervous system before the pain can be felt. The gate will only allow a certain number of messages through. If the gate can be bombarded by 'false' messages – e.g. several acupuncture needles – the gate will remain closed to the 'true' pain impulse. More specifically, it is thought that acupuncture stimulates the myelinated A-delta fibres that can close the gate to higher centres from pain information conveyed in the small, unmyelinated C fibres.
- Direct stimulation of sensory, motor and autonomic pathways causing end-organ response.
- Localized and general vasoconstriction and/or vasodilatation, increased white cell count, increased phagocytosis of leucocytes.
- Release of adrenocorticotrophic hormone and glucocorticoids (natural steroids).
- Inhibition of prostacyclin and thromboxane (factors involved in the sensation of pain).

The techniques

There are over 2000 acupuncture points, but modern practitioners often use no more than 200 of them in their day-to-day practice. The acupuncturist carefully assesses each patient and tailors treatment to the individual as a whole.

Needling
Needles finer than a hypodermic are inserted through the skin and left in for between 10–45 minutes (depending on the condition being treated). The number of needles varies but may be as few as two or three. The skin is stretched and the needles are usually inserted to a depth of 0.5–2 cm depending on the area of treatment and the patient's build. Occasionally the needles are rotated, or withdrawn and advanced alternately. Treatment may be once or twice weekly to begin with, then at longer intervals as the condition responds. Most patients return every few months for a 'top-up' session.

Acupuncturists sometimes place small ring-shaped needles (semipermanent) over the acupuncture point and hold them in place with tape to provide continuous low-level stimulation. This technique is often used when treating patients for smoking, weight loss and drug addiction. Thick, short semipermanent magnetic needles in the ear are also used by practitioners, especially for addictive disorders such as smoking, or chronic pain such as arthritis or sciatica. A patient who has the compulsion to start smoking, or who feels pain becoming intolerable, simply rubs a small magnet over the needle to re-stimulate the acupuncture point. This method of needling is rarely used now as large needles in the ear can cause bleeding under the skin with resultant necrosis (this can lead to a 'cauliflower ear').

Needles are sterile and disposable and made from stainless steel. Copper, gold, silver and platinum needles are also available but are seldom used. In certain parts of China practitioners are known to fully insert 10-cm needles straight into the abdomen – a practice not encouraged by the medical acupuncturist. However, long needles can be safely inserted parallel to the surface of the body to stimulate many adjacent points on a meridian.

The plum blossom needle is a small hammer with fine needle spikes at its head. It is used to stimulate large areas of the body by gently tapping acupuncture points. It is virtually painless and particularly useful in children.

Electroacupuncture
Many practitioners are increasingly using electroacupuncture – needles boosted by connection to a small direct current. This technique seems to work particularly well in severe pain, chronic illnesses and leg ulcers. Electroacupuncture is the most favoured form of acupuncture in Germany.

Laser acupuncture
Acupuncture points can be stimulated by a weak laser beam. The advantages of laser acupuncture are that it is completely sterile, painless and very fast.

Trigger or myofascial points
These tender points occur in muscle and fascia and can sometimes be felt as small knots. Needling these trigger points directly is often used in pain relief.

Moxibustion
Moxa wool is placed on the top of a needle and set alight. As it smoulders, heat is conducted down to the acupuncture point, increasing the strength of stimulation. Moxa sticks are also available. When lit the stick is moved up and down near the skin. Occasionally the moxa can be used directly on the skin if the patient is protected by either salt or a piece of ginger.

Cupping
Small glass cups are warmed by burning cotton wool soaked in alcohol for a few seconds inside the cup. The cup is placed over a chosen acupuncture point or points. As it cools a vacuum forms inside the cup and the underlying skin is sucked up.

Acupressure
Firm fingertip and thumb pressure on an acupuncture point will cause a short-lived effect which is particularly useful as an adjunct to traditional methods. Once patients have completed the initial 'course' of acupuncture they can be taught simple acupressure techniques until the next 'top-up' (see also 'Shiatzu' in Chapter 3).

Ear acupuncture or auriculotherapy
There are almost 300 ear acupuncture points. Most of these relate to parts of the body (Figure 2.4), and are often used in conjunction with distal acupuncture points.

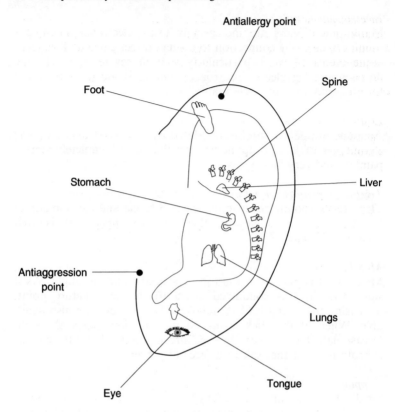

Figure 2.4 Ear acupuncture

Modern acupuncture
Modern acupuncture carried out in the UK by some NHS hospitals and by many general practitioners is based on similar principles to traditional acupuncture. However, there are a few practical differences: fewer needles are used (2–4 compared with 20–30) and they are left in for a much shorter time (occasionally less than a minute, compared with 10–45 minutes); more emphasis is placed on trigger points and on the role of nervous, immune and endocrine systems.

Traditional acupuncture
Traditional acupuncturists will also carry out tongue and pulse analysis to determine the imbalance in the flow of *chi*. A traditional diagnosis may also *sound* very different from an orthodox one.

For example, shoulder pain caused by capsulitis (inflammation of the joint) may be described as 'stagnation of *chi* in the channels around the shoulder and a *yin* deficiency'. Thrush (candidiasis) is considered a problem of 'internal damp'. A traditional acupuncturist may also advise on nutrition and lifestyle changes.

Results
A good acupuncturist can hope to help between 65% and 70% of suitable cases.

WHICH CONDITIONS ARE SUITABLE FOR TREATMENT BY ACUPUNCTURE?

- Pain relief: migraine and chronic headaches
  backache
  frozen shoulder
  bursitis
  arthritis (rheumatoid, osteoarthritis)
  gout
  repetitive strain injury
  carpal tunnel syndrome
  sports injury
  toothache
  neuralgia
  phantom limb pain
  chronic and terminal illnesses,
  e.g. multiple sclerosis, malignancy
  postoperative pain
  painful scars

- Neurological: Bell's palsy
  Ménière's disease
  vertigo

- Psychological: anxiety, panic attacks
  stress
  insomnia
  phobias
  feeling 'run down'

- Gynaecological: premenstrual tension
  menopausal symptoms
  period pain

- Urinary: Irritable or unstable bladder

- Allergies: asthma
                        hay fever
                        eczema
                        sinus and catarrhal problems

- Skin: mouth ulcers
                        chronic leg ulcers
                        pruritus
                        excessive sweating
                        psoriasis

- Abdominal: peptic ulcer
                        colitis
                        irritable bowel syndrome

- Eating disorders: compulsive eating
                        bulimia
                        anorexia

- Addictions: smoking
                        drugs (including benzodiazepines)
                        alcohol

- Bed-wetting in children

- Pregnancy: nausea and vomiting
                        labour pain

- Nausea and vomiting from anaesthesia or motion

- Tinnitus

- Twitchy eyes

- Post-viral fatigue syndrome

- Minor sports injuries

WHICH CONDITIONS ARE NOT SUITABLE FOR TREATMENT BY ACUPUNCTURE?

- Any condition that may be caused by serious underlying disease

- Bleeding tendency: patients on warfarin therapy or with bleeding disorders

- Electroacupuncture in epileptics and patients with pacemakers and cochlear implants

- Serious infections

Advantages of treatment

- Relief of pain unresponsive to conventional therapy.
- Patients often feel relaxed after therapy.
- Adjunct to conventional therapy.
- Decreased analgesic use.
- Cost-effective.
- Decreased hospital referrals.
- Relatively safe.
- Popular with the general public.
- Easily available.

Disadvantages

- Time required for adequate history, examination and needle insertion.
- Introduction of infection – human immunodeficiency virus (HIV), hepatitis, cellulitis (rare now with the use of disposable needles).
- Side-effects (rare):
  pneumothorax
  bleeding
  broken needle in situ
  light-headedness or faintness
  damage to abdominal organs.
- Occasional increase in pain after the first session ('healing crisis').

How long and how much?

First session: 30–45 minutes.
Subsequent sessions: 10–45 minutes (depending on condition).
How many sessions? Four are recommended, with regular top-up sessions every 1–6 months. If no significant change after four sessions, stop.
Cost: £25–50 per session (1996 UK prices).

NHS or private? (applicable to the UK only)

- **NHS:**
  pain clinics run by anaesthetists
  midwives at some maternity units

physiotherapists
general practitioners
certain rheumatology clinics
the Royal London Homoeopathic Hospital (if the GP has a contract with the hospital).

- **Private:** acupuncture is widely available privately, but caution is advised. Contact the organizations at the end of this chapter for authorized and/or medically qualified practitioners.

Simple self-help measures

Acupressure

Press on each point for 1–2 minutes. The location of acupressure points is given in Box 2.1.

BOX 2.1 Location of acupressure points

Bladder 23	2 fingerbreadths either side of the spine and 3 finger-breadths above the level of the upper pelvic bone (iliac crest)
Bladder 60	outside of the ankle, between the bone and Achilles tendon
Colon 4	On the back of the hand, at the end of the crease between first finger and thumb
Gallbladder 34	outside of the lower leg, below the knee joint, in front of and below the head of the fibula
Liver 2	On the top of the foot in the web between the big and second toes
Liver 3	As for Liver 2 but about 2 cm further up towards the ankle
Lung 7	2 fingerbreadths above the wrist crease on the thumb aspect
Spleen 6	4 fingerbreadths above the inside of the ankle bone, just behind the tibia
Yintang	between the eyebrows

- Migraine – Colon 4 or Liver 2.
- Sciatica – Bladder 60.
- Back pain – Bladder 23.
- Knee pain – Gallbladder 34.
- Whiplash, neck pain – Colon 4.
- Premenstrual tension – Colon 4 or Liver 3.
- Period pain – Spleen 6.
- Asthma – Colon 4 or Lung 7.
- Sinusitis – Colon 4 or Yintang.
- Stress, tension, anxiety – Colon 4 or Liver 3.
- Lethargy or fatigue – Colon 4 or Spleen 6.

Addresses for referral

British Acupuncture Association and
Register
34 Alderney Street
London SW1V 4EU
Tel. 0171 834 1012

British Acupuncture Council
Park House
206–208 Latimer Road
London W10 6RE
Tel. 0181 964 0222

British Medical Acupuncture Society
(BMAS)
Newton House
Newton Lane
Whitely
Warrington
Cheshire WA4 4JA
Tel. 01925 730727
(Doctors trained in acupuncture)

National Commission for the
Certification of Acupuncturists
1424 16th Street NW
Washington, DC 20036
USA
Tel. 202 232 1404

Royal London Homoeopathic Hospital
NHS Trust
Great Ormond Street
London WC1N 3HR
Tel. 0171 837 8833

Addresses for education and training

Academy of Chinese Acupuncture
52 Calderon Road
London E11 4EU
Tel. 0181 558 7773

British Academy of Western
Acupuncture
12 Rodney Street
Liverpool L1 2TE
Tel. 0151 709 0479
(Medical and paramedical personnel
only)

British Acupuncture Council
(Address above, will supply a list of
recognized colleges)

British Medical Acupuncture Society
(BMAS)
(Address above, doctors only)

College of Traditional Chinese
Acupuncture
Tao House
Queensway
Leamington Spa
Warwickshire CV31 3LZ
Tel. 01926 422121

London School of Acupuncture and
Traditional Chinese Medicine
3rd Floor
36 Featherstone Street
London EC1Y 8QX
Tel. 0171 490 0513
(Linked with the Register of Traditional
Chinese Medicine)

Northern College of Acupuncture
124 Acomb Road
York YO2 4EY
Tel. 01904 784828
(MSc in acupuncture, four years
part-time)

3
Manual therapies

Osteopathy and chiropractice

Background

Both osteopathy and chiropractice originate from the medically unqualified 'bonesetters' of the late nineteenth century. Osteopathy was founded by Andrew Taylor Still, an American engineer, in 1874. Still's original theories were gleaned from his personal and religious convictions. He was convinced that the body tended towards health and had within it its own medicine. Man became ill if the body's structure became maladjusted causing a reduction in arterial circulation. If the body could be re-adjusted it would again work perfectly. In 1917 these concepts were brought to the UK by Martin Littlejohn, founder of the British School of Osteopathy. He called osteopathy the 'science of adjustment'.

It was an osteopath and healer, D. D. Palmer, who laid down the principles of chiropractice in 1895. He cured a patient who had been suffering from deafness by manipulating some malaligned vertebrae in his neck. Palmer reasoned that small displacements of the spinal column interfered with nerve impulses causing abnormal function.

Modern osteopathy and chiropractice apply themselves to the body's biomechanical problems. The view is that the pain and disability affecting a sufferer stem from a flaw in the function of the musculoskeletal system rather than an obvious pathological cause. These flaws can exist without symptoms but may throw excessive strain on another part of the body.

Research

- Meade, T. W., Dyer, S., Browne, W. *et al.* (1990). Low back pain of mechanical origin. A randomized comparison of chiropractice and hospital outpatient treatment. *British Medical Journal*, **300**: 1431–7.
- Koes, B. W., Bouter, L. M., van Mameren, H. *et al.* (1992).

Randomized clinical trial of manipulative therapy and physiotherapy for persistent back and neck complaints: results of one-year follow-up. *British Medical Journal*, **304**(6827): 601–5.

Both of these well-respected studies showed that chiropractic therapy for lower back pain is more effective than hospital physiotherapy or treatment by a general practitioner.

● Anderson, R., Meeker, W. C., Wirick, B. E. *et al.* (1992). A meta-analysis of clinical trials of spinal manipulation. *Journal of Manipulative and Physiological Therapeutics*, **15**(3): 181–94.

A review of 23 randomized controlled trials showed that spinal manipulation was more effective than any comparable treatment such as physiotherapy.

Mechanism of action

Osteopathy and chiropractice are now firmly a part of the 'new orthodoxies' (including acupuncture and homoeopathy). Their aim is to realign the body and to mobilize joints and connective tissue. Doing so restores movement in restricted joints, reduces the strain on other joints and improves mobility and general health.

Despite relatively little research, some theories have been put forward to explain the basis of these disciplines:

● Musculoskeletal displacements or flaws can be caused by stresses, strains (e.g. sudden exertion), accidents or congenital skeletal abnormalities. Bad posture or incorrect use can place uneven or excessive loads on the musculoskeletal system.
● Defects or displacements in joints may affect surrounding muscles, ligaments and nerves. Biochemical function may also be affected.
● Pain and restricted movement may be caused by distortion of the joint cartilage and capsule, or ligament stretching. These changes are not visible on X-ray but may produce symptoms directly or by their effects on nerve stimulation.
● Persistent irritation may affect internal viscera (e.g. lungs, stomach) by interfering with electrical nerve impulses, chemical neurotransmitters or other materials that may flow along the nerve.
● Prolonged rest may cause a gradual loss of mechanoreceptor activity. This in turn may alter the central interaction between these receptors and nerves which selectively respond to pain (nociceptors). Stimulation of these mechanoreceptors by manipulation, traction or vibration can alleviate pain.

The techniques

The practitioner will begin by recording a full medical history of the problem including trauma, injuries and past treatments.

Examination of posture and palpation of the vertebral column at rest and on passive and active movements are always carried out ('motion palpation'). The practitioner looks for excessive mobility or (more usually) a lack of mobility. Straight leg raising, muscle assessment, leg measurement and routine neurological tests may also be carried out if indicated. Chiropractors tend to use X-rays for diagnosis, whereas osteopaths use X-rays more as a back-up measure to confirm findings made on palpation.

Some of the specialist techniques used are described below.

High-velocity manipulation
An area of displacement will usually be manipulated back into position. The body may be placed in awkward positions enabling it to be used as a long lever. Skilful manipulation is quick (high-velocity) and pain-free with very short joint movement. Often there is an accompanying crack or clunk. Such long-lever techniques allow the vertebra to right itself and often require minimal force from the practitioner. Compare this with low-velocity mobilization done by doctors and physiotherapists where the joint remains within its passive range of motion.

Direct-thrust manipulation
Direct thrusts involve placing pressure on the affected vertebra and using a specific push to reposition it. A loud clunk may also be heard, often accompanied by instant relief.

Springing
Springing is used to provide shearing forces to improve mobility between joints which do not normally have a wide range of movement, e.g. the sacroiliac joints.

Articulation
Articulation involves repeated rhythmical manoeuvres which take the joints through their normal range of movement. It can be extremely effective in restoring normal joint function and alleviating pain by stretching muscles and ligaments and encouraging joint surfaces to move in their correct position.

Joint release
The affected joint is taken to the extreme of its range of movement.
The practitioner then applies a steady force to the joint causing it to
'unlock' or 'release'.

Massage
Massage is used to treat tense muscle groups or to relax tissues that
may surround another problem, e.g. a prolapsed disc. Various
stretching, kneading and rolling movements are made with the
hands and fingers; the aim is also to stimulate the circulation and
drain lymphatics. Localized tender spots (trigger points) can be
specifically targeted. Massage is also used as a preliminary technique to ready the body for manipulation.

Cranial osteopathy
Sometimes called 'fluid osteopathy', cranial osteopathy was first
described by William Garner Sutherland in 1899. He postulated
that gentle manual compression and tapping of the skull could
improve the circulation of cerebrospinal fluid. Although this technique has few advocates at present it is gaining more acceptance,
particularly in the treatment of children under 5 years of age.
Some of the conditions treated include birth trauma, autism, spas-
ticity and hyperactivity.

McTimoney technique
McTimoney chiropractice came about as a result of a split in
the chiropractic movement. Practitioners of this therapy consider
it a more faithful version of original chiropractice. The essential
difference is that the McTimoney technique uses a more gentle
approach.

Prescribed exercises
At the end of the session the practitioner may demonstrate certain
specific exercises to be carried out at home. These help to maintain
mobility until the next treatment. Advice may also be given on
posture, work positions and methods of relaxing. Some practitioners are also naturopaths and will advise on diet and general
nutrition.

WHICH CONDITIONS ARE SUITABLE FOR TREATMENT BY OSTEOPATHY OR CHIROPRACTICE?

- Back pain:
  acute (under 3 weeks) **uncomplicated**
  e.g. disc prolapse, central stenosis, lateral stenosis, spondylolisthesis, segmental instability, sacroiliac strain, simple mechanical back pain
  acute with minor neurological findings
  e.g. asymmetrical decreased ankle reflex, minor sensory loss, normal X-rays
  acute back pain in pregnancy
  chronic pain (when organic causes excluded)

- Upper and lower limb joint pain and stiffness
  e.g. strains, dislocations, non-specific pain

- Upper and lower limb muscular pain and stiffness

- Whiplash injuries

- Brachial neuritis

- Migraine

- Cluster headaches

- Cervical and tension headaches

- Benign paroxysmal positional vertigo

- Repetitive strain injury (RSI)

- Tennis or golfer's elbow

- Carpal tunnel syndrome

- Sports injuries

- Sinus and catarrh problems

WHICH CONDITIONS ARE NOT SUITABLE FOR TREATMENT BY OSTEOPATHY OR CHIROPRACTICE?

- Any condition that may be caused by serious underlying disease

- A previous unfavourable response to manipulation

- Acute or unhealed fractures

- Ligament laxity or injury (instability)

- Rheumatoid arthritis

- Advanced ankylosing spondylitis
- Bone disease, e.g. secondary spread from a cancer
- Serious infections
- Disc prolapse with progressive neurological signs
- Severe osteoporosis
- Bleeding tendency, e.g. warfarin therapy or a bleeding disorder
- History of transient ischaemic attacks (TIAs)
- Vascular insufficiency of the vertebral artery

Advantages

- Adjunct to conventional therapy.
- Occasionally give immediate pain relief.
- Often more effective than physiotherapy.
- Decrease in medication.
- Earlier return to work for many back-pain sufferers.
- Safe.
- Cost-effective.

Disadvantages

- Cost usually borne by patient.
- Patients often self-refer. An underlying organic condition may be inappropriately treated by an inexperienced practitioner.
- Occasional discomfort after treatment.
- Rarely, pain becomes worse.
- Vascular accidents causing stroke from cervical manipulation – extremely rare (1 in 10 million).

How long and how much?

First appointment: 45 minutes to 1 hour.
Subsequent appointments: 20–40 minutes.
How many sessions? Three to eight sessions depending on ailment, with occasional follow-up treatments.
Cost: £25–40 per session (1996 UK prices).

NHS or private? (applicable to the UK only)

- **NHS:** osteopathy and chiropractice are practised by few doctors. However, with the advent of fundholding in the UK many general practitioners are 'buying in' osteopathy services on a private basis – where available this is free to the patient.
- **Private:** widely available privately. Many practitioners work out of natural health clinics. Many patients take advice from their general practitioner. Refer only to members of the relevant professional organization.

Addresses for referral

American Chiropractic Association
1701 Clarendon Blvd
Arlington, VA 22209
USA
Tel. 800 986 4636

American Osteopathic Association
142 East Ontario Street
Chicago, IL 60611
USA
Tel. 312 280 5800

British Chiropractic Association
29 Whitely Street
Reading
Berks RG2 0EG
Tel. 01734 757557

General Council and Register of
Osteopaths
56 London Street
Reading
Berkshire RG1 4SQ
Tel. 01734 576585

Osteopathic Information Service
PO Box 2074
Reading RG1 4YR
Tel. 01734 512051

Scottish Chiropractic Association
30 Roseburn Place
Edinburgh EH12 5NX
Tel. 0131 346 7500

Addresses for education and training

Anglo-European College of
Chiropractice
13–15 Parkwood Road
Boscombe
Bournemouth
Dorset BH5 2DF
Tel. 01202 436200
(Five-year BSc course; graduates of the AECC are eligible to become members of the British Chiropractic Association)

British College of Naturopathy and
Osteopathy
Frazer House
6 Netherall Gardens
London NW3 5RR
Tel. 0171 435 7830

British Institute of Musculoskeletal
Medicine
27 Green Lane
Northwood
Middlesex HA6 2PX
Tel. 01923 820110
(Doctors only; regular 2-day and 5-day courses)

British Osteopathic Association
8–10 Boston Place
London NW1 6QH
Tel. 0171 262 5250
(Admits doctors only)

British School of Osteopathy
1–4 Suffolk Street
London SW1Y 4HG
Tel. 0171 930 9254
(Four years full-time)

Applied kinesiology

Background

Kinesiology means 'the study of motion or movement'. Applied kinesiology (AK) was first devised by an American chiropractor, Dr George J. Goodheart, in 1964. He discovered that testing muscle strength and tone could reveal specific information about a patient's health and the state of the internal organs.

The system is an amalgamation of general chiropractic anatomy and techniques and the meridian theory of acupuncture. Certain muscle groups are related to internal organs by the meridians that pass over them, for example the muscles surrounding the shoulder are linked to the liver, and the hamstrings are similarly 'connected' to the large intestine. Once a diagnosis has been made treatment is given by manipulation and massage. 'Touch for health' is a simplified form of AK, devised in the early 1970s by John Thie, for use by individuals in their own home.

The use of kinesiology in the detection of allergies, vitamin and mineral deficiencies and the concept of electromagnetic fields and surrogate testees (see below) has brought considerable controversy into this form of complementary medicine. However, AK is becoming increasingly popular worldwide amongst osteopaths and chiropractors, especially those involved in sports medicine.

Research

There has been very little serious research carried out into AK. Much published information is anecdotal.

Mechanism of action

Practitioners, like traditional acupuncturists, believe that stress, trauma and disease can cause an imbalance of internal energy or *chi* in related body organs and muscles. Kinesiology re-balances the *chi* and promotes health.

Some also believe that an abnormal electromagnetic field exists around the patient which can be detected by the kinesiologist.

The techniques

There are over 40 specific muscle tests that can be carried out during an examination. Typically the patient extends an arm which the practitioner tries to push down using light pressure for a few seconds. If the arm 'locks' in this position it indicates strength and health in the shoulder muscles. However, if the arm feels heavy to the patient, starts to shake or feels 'spongy' then a weakness may be present. More specfic tests are then carried out to identify the individual muscles affected.

Once weakness has been picked up the affected group of muscles is re-balanced to restore *chi* and effect recovery. For example, constipation may be caused by an energy imbalance in the hamstrings. Massaging the hamstrings may improve the constipation. Massage is often concentrated on the areas overlying origins and insertions of muscles.

Kinesiology is also used to detect allergies and nutritional needs. If an allergen is placed in the patient's mouth or held near the skin, muscular weakness may develop. This technique is being increasingly used in America by dentists to assess sensitivity to mercury amalgam fillings.

Examination of children and patients too ill to co-operate may be carried out through a 'surrogate testee'.

Energy is transferred to the surrogate from the patient by touch. The kinesiologist then examines the surrogate, makes a diagnosis and treats the patient.

WHICH CONDITIONS ARE SUITABLE FOR TREATMENT BY KINESIOLOGY?

- Specific allergies, latent food allergies
- Backache
- Neck pain
- Generalized stiffness and aches
- Tiredness and malaise
- Skin problems
- Sinus problems
- Depression
- Anxiety
- Phobias
- Sports injuries
- Irritable bowel syndrome
- Migraine, headaches

WHICH CONDITIONS ARE NOT SUITABLE FOR TREATMENT BY KINESIOLOGY?

- Any condition that may be caused by serious underlying disease
- Scar tissue
- Infectious diseases
- Inflammation or infection of veins or lymphatics
- Deep vein thrombosis
- Shingles

Advantages

- Helps with many niggling problems that can lead to disease.
- Non-invasive.
- Safe.

Disadvantages

- Not available on the NHS.
- Cost borne by patient.
- Still relatively few experienced practitioners.
- A large element of controversy in its techniques and mechanism of action.

How long and how much?

First session: up to 1 hour.
Subsequent sessions: 15–20 minutes.
How many sessions? Four to six sessions. If no better, stop and consult your doctor.
Cost: £25–40 per session (1996 UK prices).

NHS or private? (applicable to the UK only)

Kinesiology is not available on the NHS.

Addresses for referral

Association of Systematic Kinesiology
39 Browns Road
Surbiton
Surrey KT5 8ST
Tel. 0181 399 3215

Kinesiology Federation
PO Box 7891
Wimbledon
London SW19 1ZB
Tel. 0181 545 0255

Addresses for education and training

Association of Systematic Kinesiology
(address above)

International College of Applied
Kinesiology
PO Box 680547
Park City, Utah 84068
USA
Tel. 913 542 1801
(For doctors and chiropractors only)

International Kinesiology College
Lehenstrasse 36
Zurich
Switzerland CH 8037

Touch for Health Foundation
1174 North Lake Avenue
Pasadena, CA 91104–3797
USA
Tel. 818 794 1181

Reflexology

Background

Reflexology (or 'zone therapy') aims to treat the whole body through contact with the feet. Its use was widespread in ancient civilizations including the Japanese, Indians, Egyptians and, inevitably, the Chinese 5000 years ago. Modern reflexology owes its origins to an American ear, nose and throat specialist Dr William Fitzgerald, who in the 1920s was able to carry out minor ear operations after anaesthetizing an area by pressure on a part of the foot. The concept was extended in the USA by the physiotherapist Eunice Ingham. She originated the first maps which charted the body onto the feet. Doreen Bayly, a student of Ingham, introduced reflexology to the UK in the early 1960s.

There are areas or 'reflexes' in the feet that represent all parts of the body (Figures 3.1 and 3.2). These reflexes are found on the sole, side and top of each foot. The right and left feet represent corresponding areas of the body from the 'top down'. Thus the toes represent the brain and sinuses, the digestive tract is in the middle of the foot and the heel represents the genitalia. Similar reflexes are found in the hand, but the feet are preferred because they are more sensitive and the reflex areas are larger.

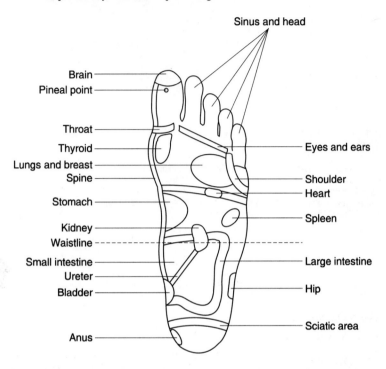

Figure 3.1 Reflexes of the left foot (sole)

Research

There has been no published evidence of the effectiveness of reflexology.

Mechanism of action

Some of the traditionally held beliefs are:

- Massage improves blood and lymph circulation to the corresponding part of the body.
- Therapy decreases nervous tension around the affected area and re-activates the body's natural healing ability.
- Crystalline deposits may be present in certain reflex areas. The deposits feel like granules and are thought to interfere with nerve impulses. Massage clears the problem by breaking down the crystals and promoting nerve transmission.

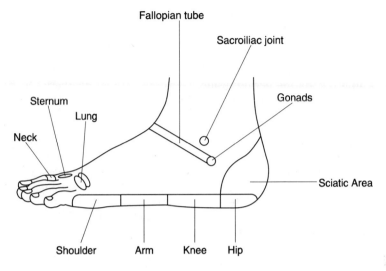

Figure 3.2 Reflexes of the left foot (dorsal)

The techniques

Initial assessment

After giving a full history of the problem, the patient reclines with the knees slightly flexed and the feet usually on the practitioner's lap. The reflexologist will then examine the feet, noting any signs of infection, the presence of hard skin, corns, verrucae, the state of the nails, scars or injuries, swelling, temperature, colour and perspiration. The feet are readied by a gentle massage using talcum powder.

The thumb is held bent and the side and end of the thumb are used to apply firm pressure on a reflex point, which can be no bigger than a pinhead. 'Creeping' movements are used to move from one reflex to the next to avoid loss of contact with the foot.

Some areas may feel very tender. The sensation may vary from a sharp pain to a dull ache. Reflexologists believe that pain occurs in areas of energy blockage. Treatment relieves this blockage and eventually the pain. Both feet are treated.

Patients are often given hand reflexology techniques to practise on themselves until the next session.

Cross reflexes

Cross reflexes are links between the joints of the body on the same side, i.e. the shoulder with the hip, elbow and knee, and wrist and ankle. For example, tenderness in the elbow may be relieved by massaging a tender point in the knee.

Metamorphic technique

This offshoot of reflexology considers the foot representative of the 9-month gestation period inside the womb. A light, feathery touch is used to help emotional problems developed during this time. Particularly useful in mentally and physically handicapped children.

Vacuflex reflexology

Vacuflex therapy was introduced to the UK in the late 1980s after initial development in South Africa. It is a bi-phasic treatment using foot reflexes and acupuncture meridians. It is ideal for patients who cannot tolerate finger pressure in conventional reflexology. Felt boots are placed over the feet from which air is sucked out to form a vacuum. This uniformly stimulates all the reflexes. Coloured patterns remain on the feet after the boots are removed which last for 15–20 seconds. These relate to areas of congestion and infection in the body. These patterns change after each treatment and can illustrate progress made during and after treatment. The second stage of each treatment involves the stimulation of meridians which run across the feet, legs, hands and arms (see Figure 2.3). Silicone pads are used instead of needles and are kept in place by a gentle vacuum.

WHICH CONDITIONS ARE SUITABLE FOR TREATMENT BY REFLEXOLOGY?

- Musculoskeletal: back pain
                      neck pain
                      stiff or painful joints

- Psychological: depression
                      insomnia
                      anxiety
                      stress
                      loss of libido
                      post-natal depression
                      feeling 'run down', exhausted

- Gynaecological: heavy, painful periods
                      premenstrual tension
                      menopausal symptoms

- Obstetric: labour pains

- Asthma
- Hay fever
- Sinusitis
- Eczema
- Migraine
- Tension headaches
- Restless legs
- Addictions: alcohol
                        smoking
                        chocolate
- Progressive disorders: multiple sclerosis
                                     Parkinson's disease
- Post-viral fatigue syndrome

WHICH CONDITIONS ARE NOT SUITABLE FOR TREATMENT BY REFLEXOLOGY?

- Any condition that may be caused by serious underlying disease
- Infectious diseases
- Inflammation or infection of veins or lymphatics
- Deep vein thrombosis
- Shingles
- Severe fungal infection of the feet
- Psychiatric patients on high-dose drugs

Advantages
- Gentle, non-invasive.
- Safe.
- Most patients feel calm and revitalized after treatment.
- Popular with the general public.
- Portable skill.

Disadvantages

- Not usually available on the NHS.
- Cost borne by patient.
- Some patients may suffer from a 'healing crisis' after a treatment as the body fights to eliminate 'toxins'. The symptoms are usually short-lived but can include:
    fatigue
    change in sleep pattern
    increased urination
    increased bowel activity
    increased perspiration
    increased vaginal discharge
    coughing, sneezing
- Research needs to be carried out on the underlying rationale of therapy.
- Not suitable for those with a 'ticklish' disposition.

How long and how much?

First session: up to 1 hour.
Subsequent sessions: 30 minutes.
How many sessions? Results should be evident after three treatments; a course of six to eight sessions is usually recommended.
Cost: £20–25 (1996 UK prices).

NHS or private? (applicable to the UK only)

- **NHS:** some GP practices have brought in reflexology with fund-holding but this is uncommon. Midwives occasionally give reflexology for pain relief in labour or post-natal depression.
- **Private:** widely available privately. Many work out of natural health clinics. Some therapists will do home visits. Refer only to members of professional organizations.

Addresses for referral

British Complementary Medicine
Association
9 Soar Lane
Leicester LE3 5DE
Tel. 01162 425406

British Register of Complementary
Practitioners
Reflexology Division
PO Box 194
London SE16 1QZ
Tel. 0171 237 5165

Holistic Healing Centre
92 Sheering Road
Old Harlow
Essex CM17 0JW
Tel. 01279 429060

Reflexologists Society
Membership Secretary
135 Collins Meadow
Harlow
Essex CM19 4EJ

Metamorphic Association
New Cross Natural Therapy Centre
67 Ritherdon Road
London SW17 8QE
Tel. 0181 672 5951

Addresses for education and training

Most courses are part-time or weekends only.

British Complementary Medicine
Association
(address above)

Holistic Healing Centre
(address above)

British School for Reflex Zone Therapy
of the Feet
97 Oakington Avenue
Wembley Park
London HA9 8HY
Tel. 0181 908 2201
(Doctors and nurses only)

Midland School of Reflex Therapy
5 Church Street
Warwick CB34 4AS
Tel. 01926 491071

Shiatzu

Background

Shiatzu evolved from ancient Chinese massage, and like its ancestor involves the concepts of internal energy (*chi*), *yin* and *yang* and acupuncture meridians. As such there is little difference between shiatzu and acupressure. Indeed many practitioners use the terms synonomously. Shiatzu is still commonly practised in Japan (a profession often chosen by the blind), where it is seen by many as a form of preventative health and self-treatment.

Research

There have been no controlled trials on the benefits of shiatzu *per se*. However, its mechanism of action and beneficial effects are similar to needle acupuncture. Some of the research carried out on acupuncture could reasonably be extrapolated to shiatzu.

Mechanism of action

The explanation of shiatzu (and acupressure) lies almost totally in Chinese theory. Re-balancing *chi* that may be overactive, stagnant or weak allows the body to repair itself and maintain good health.

There is transference of healing energy from masseur to patient during the process of touch. Massage itself improves circulation of blood and lymph, breaks down adhesions and relaxes muscles. (See also Chapter 2.)

The techniques

Practitioners aim to gain a better understanding of the patient's condition by looking and touching after taking a full medical and personal history. Some may also carry out pulse and tongue diagnosis.

The patient lies on a mat on the floor; occasionally treatment can be given to patients seated in a chair. Constant fingertip pressure is applied to various acupuncture points. On larger areas pressure may be applied using hands, elbows or feet. Herbs and oils may be used to augment treatment.

Specific pressure techniques are used to 'calm', 'tonify' or 'disperse' *chi*. If *chi* is overactive it can be calmed by using the palm of the hand to cover the acupuncture point or apply very light pressure (by gentle stroking) to the area. Weak *chi* can be tonified by applying stationary firm pressure perpendicular to the acupuncture point. A circular motion or 'pumping' in and out will disperse stagnant *chi*. Warming the acupuncture point by holding a lighted moxa or incense stick 2 cm above the area will also allow tonification.

Practitioners enhance their techniques by 'opening' meridians and bringing them nearer the surface. This is achieved by placing the arms and legs of the patient in certain positions for a few minutes at a time.

Jin shen do is a subtle form of shiatzu where holding or a slight pulling action is preferred. *Shen tao* acupressure involves lighter finger pressure over acupuncture points.

At the end of a session the practitioner may recommend exercises and dietary and lifestyle changes.

WHICH CONDITIONS ARE SUITABLE FOR TREATMENT BY SHIATZU?

- Musculoskeletal:
  back pain
  neck pain
  arthritis
  aching joints
  muscle stiffness
  cramps
  carpal tunnel syndrome

- Minor sports injuries

- Psychological:
  anxiety
  stress
  insomnia
  depression
  poor libido
  feeling 'run down'

- Allergies:
  asthma
  hay fever
  sinus and catarrhal problems

- Gynaecological:
  painful periods
  premenstrual tension
  menopausal symptoms

- Headaches, migraine

- Post-viral fatigue syndrome

- Restless legs

- Jet-lag

- Nausea and vomiting

- Diarrhoea

- Influenza and colds

- Irritable bowel syndrome

- Progressive conditions: multiple sclerosis
  Parkinson's disease

WHICH CONDITIONS ARE NOT SUITABLE FOR TREATMENT BY SHIATZU?

- Any condition that may be caused by serious underlying disease.
- Early pregnancy (before 3 months)
- Sexually transmitted diseases
- Infectious diseases
- Inflammation or infection of veins or lymphatics
- Deep vein thrombosis
- Shingles
- Scar tissue

Advantages

- Gentle, non-invasive.
- Safe.
- Many patients feel relaxed and invigorated after treatment.

Disadvantages

- Not usually available on the NHS.
- Cost borne by patient.
- Some patients may suffer from a 'healing crisis' after the first few treatments as toxins are released. Headaches and flu-like symptoms may occur for up to 24 hours.
- Scepticism surrounds its Chinese philosophy.

How long and how much?

First session: 1 hour.
Subsequent sessions: 40–50 minutes.
How many sessions? Four to six recommended. Patients often continue indefinitely to help relaxation.
Cost: £20–35 per session (1996 UK prices). Most therapists offer a sliding scale of fees.

NHS or private? (applicable to the UK only)

- **NHS:** acupressure is available at St Thomas's Hospital, London. More NHS treatment may be available in hospital pain clinics in the future.
- **Private:** widely available. Many therapists work out of natural health clinics or from home. Refer only to members of professional bodies.

Address for referral

Shiatzu Society
5 Foxcote
Wokingham
Berks RG11 3PG
Tel. 01734 730836

Addresses for education and training

British School of Shiatzu
6 Erskine Road
London SE3 3EJ
Tel. 0171 483 3776

Jin Shen Do Foundation
PO Box 1097
Felton, CA 95018
USA
Tel. 408 338 9454

Middle Piccadilly Natural Healing Centre
Holwell
Nr Sherborne
Dorset DT9 5LW
Tel. 01963 23468
(3 year part-time course for Shen Tao)

Rolfing

Background

Rolfing or 'structural integration' was first developed by Dr Ida Rolf (1896–1979) who used this technique of deep massage long before the establishment of the Rolf Institute in Boulder, Colorado in 1973. The basis of action is the supposition that stresses and strains imposed on our bodies owing to poor posture, injury and the force of gravity, cause musculoskeletal imbalance and asymmetry. To overcome these structural problems rolfing works, not by curing, but by altering, correcting and re-educating the body.

Research

There have been no controlled studies of the benefits of rolfing.

Mechanism of action

Deep massage and pressure is used to break up muscular scar tissue and adhesions. It also softens up other tissues in the body (ligaments, tendons and fascia) to free them up from fixed or inefficient positions and postures.

Realigning the body so that 'gravity can flow' more easily helps reduce the stresses and strains imposed on it by poor posture and injury.

All the moving parts of the body interact. If one part of the 'machinery' is defective it will affect the efficiency of the whole system.

The techniques

A full medical history is taken with particular emphasis on operations and musculoskeletal injuries.

The body is assessed from all perspectives (back, front, sitting, walking, lying, etc.) to see how its structure and function integrate. Some practitioners will take 'before and after' photographs to allow comparison and monitor effects of treatment.

By using fingers, hands, elbows and knees, deep massage and pressure are given to specific areas of the body at each of the initial five or six sessions. Deep massage can be painful and patients are encouraged to let their emotions out by crying out or groaning. The patient is asked to assist therapy by breathing and moving in certain ways on the rolfer's instruction.

During the following four or five sessions the now more flexible tissues are re-educated and each structural system in the body is encouraged to work with the next.

Prescribed exercises
Specific exercises are given to the patient to carry out at home until the next follow-up session.

Hellerwork
Hellerwork is a gentler form of rolfing with an almost psycho-therapeutic approach to the thoughts and emotions released during therapy. Emphasis is also put on movement education.

Aston patterning
Movement education and gentle massage are the mainstays of Aston patterning treatment.

WHICH CONDITIONS ARE SUITABLE FOR TREATMENT BY ROLFING?

- Chronic structural problems: back pain
  - neck pain
  - stiff or painful joints
  - poor posture

- Any activity or occupation where a body in optimum condition is important, e.g. athletes, dancers, musicians

- Occasionally used as an adjunct to psychotherapy

WHICH CONDITIONS ARE NOT SUITABLE FOR TREATMENT BY ROLFING?

- Any condition that may be caused by serious underlying disease

- Early pregnancy (before 3 months)

- Sexually transmitted diseases

- Infectious diseases

- Inflammation or infection of veins or lymphatics

- Deep vein thrombosis

- Shingles

- Scar tissue

- Varicose veins

Advantages

- Non-invasive.
- Safe.
- Patients can often experience positive emotional changes.

Disadvantages

- Not available on the NHS.
- More costly than other complementary techniques (ten sessions required).
- Few practitioners generally available.

How long and how much?

First session: $1\frac{1}{2}$ hours.
Subsequent sessions: $1-1\frac{1}{2}$ hours.
How many sessions? Ten are recommended, ideally spaced at one to three per week. A specific part of the body is treated at each session. Practitioners emphasize the gradual nature of rolfing.
Cost: £50–60 per session (1996 UK prices).

NHS or private? (applicable to the UK only)

Rolfing is not available on the NHS.

Addresses for referral and education

Aston Training Center
PO Box 544
Mill Valley, CA 94941
USA
Tel. 702 831 8228

Bodyworkers
Suite 211
Coppergate House
16 Brune Street
London E1 7NJ
Tel. 0171 721 7833
(for Hellerwork)

European Rolfing Association
Ohmstrasse 9
80802 München
Germany

Rolf Institute
80 Clifton Hill
London NW8 0JT
Tel. 0171 328 9026

Rolf Institute
205 Canyon Boulevard
Boulder, CO 80302
USA
Tel. 303 449 5903

Rolfing
Ms Jenny Crewdson
Tel. 0171 834 1493

Massage

Background

Massage is an effective manual therapy that has been used in the ancient cultures of India, Persia, China, Arabia, Egypt and Greece. Although there are over 80 different types of massage recognized today, most modern techniques are derived from Per Henrik Ling's (1776–1839) practice of Swedish or 'classical' massage.

Massage is often used in conjunction with other therapies (e.g. osteopathy, polarity, aromatherapy, rolfing, reflexology, shiatzu and kinesiology) and is currently enjoying re-emergence as a therapy in itself after trying to shake off the massage-parlour image.

Research

There have been many good studies of massage over the years which have shown definite therapeutic benefits.

- de Brujin, R. (1984). Deep transverse friction, it's analgesic effect. *International Journal of Sports Medicine*, **5**: 35–6.

A few minutes of friction massage relieved pain from 20 seconds to 48 hours.

- Li, Z. M. (1984). 235 cases of frozen shoulder treated by manipulation and massage. *Journal of Traditional Chinese Medicine*, **4**: 213–5.

In this study, 205 patients who had gradual stretching and massage improved in their range of movement and pain levels, and 71% recovered completely. Of the 30 who had manipulation under anesthaesia, only a third improved with 10% going on to complete cure.

- Field, T. M., Schanberg, S. M., Scafidi, F. *et al.* (1986). Tactile/kinesthetic stimulation effects on preterm neonates. *Pediatrics*, **77**(5): 654–8.

Twenty premature neonates were stroked for three 10-minute periods daily for 10 days. These babies gained 47% more weight per day, showed more developed behaviour, were more alert and active and left hospital an average of 6 days earlier than babies who had not received the tactile stimulation.

- Field, T., Morrow, C., Valdeon, C. *et al.* (1992). Massage reduces anxiety in child and adolescent psychiatric patients.

Journal of the American Academy of Child and Adolescent Psychiatry, **31**(1): 125–31.

A half-an-hour massage a day reduced anxiety and depression more than a relaxing videotape.

- Ferrell-Torry, A. T. and Glick, O. J. (1993). The use of therapeutic massage as a nursing intervention to modify anxiety and perception of cancer pain. *Cancer Nursing*, **16**(2): 93–101.

Pain perception was reduced by 60% and anxiety levels by 24% in cancer patients receiving massage.

Mechanism of action

- Massage

  eases muscle tension
  relaxes knotted tissue
  stretches scar tissue
  breaks down adhesions
  increases blood and lymph circulation

  The psychological benefits of 'massage touch' undoubtedly contribute to its therapeutic effect.

The techniques

Ideally massage should be carried out on a firm couch and at a comfortable room temperature. Basic carrier oils (e.g. almond or olive oil) or talcum powder can be used. Swedish massage is the most commonly practised form of massage therapy. It incorporates four basic techniques:

Effleurage
Effleurage consists of slow, gliding strokes using the palms, fingertips and ball of the thumb. Deeper massage can be given using knuckles or thumbs.

Percussion or tapotement
Sharp, fast, stimulating movements are used to tone and strengthen muscles. Movements are usually delivered with the side of the hand or fingers and include cupping, hacking ('karate chop') and clapping.

Friction or frottage
Deep massage by a series of small circular movements, using the
thumbs, fingers or heel of the hand, helps ease muscle tension
and improve blood and lymph circulation.

Pétrissage
Deep, vigorous, sometimes painful massage by kneading and
squeezing between finger and thumb (like a baker with dough),
helps to relax muscles and improve circulation.

**WHICH CONDITIONS ARE SUITABLE FOR TREATMENT
BY MASSAGE?**

- Musculoskeletal: back pain
    neck pain
    arthritis
    aching joints
    muscle stiffness
    cramps

- Minor sports injuries: soft tissue injuries

- Psychological: anxiety
    stress
    insomnia
    depression
    feeling 'run down'

- Gynaecological: premenstrual tension

- Headaches

- Post-viral fatigue syndrome

- Restless legs

- Jet-lag

- Irritable bowel syndrome

- Progressive conditions: multiple sclerosis
    Parkinson's disease

- Terminal disease: cancers

WHICH CONDITIONS ARE NOT SUITABLE FOR TREATMENT BY MASSAGE?

- Any condition that may be caused by serious underlying disease
- Early pregnancy (before 3 months)
- Sexually transmitted diseases
- Infectious diseases
- Inflammation or infection of veins or lymphatics
- Deep vein thrombosis
- Shingles
- Scar tissue
- Varicose veins

Advantages

- Non-invasive.
- Safe.
- Patients can often experience positive emotional changes.
- Easy to learn the basics.
- Very little equipment is needed.
- Increasing in popularity with the general public.

Disadvantages

- Time and cost may be prohibitive for some.
- Poor technique may cause repetitive strain injury in the masseur.
- Massage-parlour image still exists.

How long and how much?

First session: 45 minutes to $1\frac{1}{2}$ hours.
Subsequent sessions: 1 hour.
How many sessions? Occasionally only one. Many clients return for regular therapy.
Cost: £25–50 per session (1996 UK prices).

NHS or private? (applicable to the UK only)

- **NHS:** massage is being increasingly used in cancer patients as an adjunct to pain and anxiety management. Many physio-therapists, nurses and midwives are learning massage to augment their own clinical skills.
- **Private:** widely available in gymnasiums and fitness clubs. Basic courses are available locally, often in adult education centres.

Addresses for referral

American Massage Therapy Association
820 Davis Street
Evanston, IL 60201
USA
Tel. 708 864 0123

Clare Maxwell Hudson School of
Massage
PO Box 457
London NW2 4BR
Tel. 0181 450 6494

Fellowship of Sports Masseurs and
Therapists
BM Soigneur
London WC1N 3XX
Tel. 0181 886 3120

London and Counties Society of
Physiologists
100 Waterloo Road
Blackpool FY4 1AW
Tel. 01253 408443

Addresses for training and education

Churchill Centre
22 Montague Street
London W1H 1TB
Tel. 0171 402 9475

Clare Maxwell Hudson School of
Massage
(address above)

College of Holistic Medicine
4 Craigpark
Glasgow G31 2NA
Tel. 0141 554 5808

Dancing Dragon School
115 Manor Road
London N16 5PB
Tel. 0181 800 0471

London School of Sports Massage
88 Cambridge Street
London SW1V 4QG
Tel. 0171 234 5962

Northern Institute of Massage
100 Waterloo Road
Blackpool
Lancs FY4 1AW
Tel. 01253 403548

Retford International College
Storcroft House
London Road
Retford
Nottingham DN22 7EB
Tel. 01777 707371

Polarity

Background

A system of balancing energy flow, polarity therapy was devised by an American osteopath and naturopath Dr Randolph Stone (1890–1983). His research for a universal system of medical treatment led him to incorporate the Western theories of osteopathy with the Eastern theories of yoga and ayurveda. Stone postulated that life is energy that flows cyclically from positive to neutral to negative and back again. He used the Eastern concepts of *chakras* (see Figure 7.1) and the 'five element system' to describe the presence and flow of this energy or *prana*. *Chakras* are foci in the body through which energies flow and help maintain physical and psychological make-up. The element system proposes that an individual is made up of five representative states: fire, ether, air, earth and water. In Chinese philosophy the ether and air elements are replaced by metal and wood. Each of the elements represents different body organs. Every organ is linked by this element system and can affect and be affected by positive or negative energy flow from other organs.

By picking up the quality, nature and location of energy imbalance in the *chakras* and elements a therapist can diagnose the nature of the patient's ailment.

Research

Although much research has been carried out on related techniques such as massage and osteopathy, none has concentrated specifically on polarity therapy.

Mechanism of action

Except for a central neutral energy core, all points in the body are either positive or negative. For example, the head and right hand are positive, whereas the soles of the feet and the left hand are negative. Ailments are caused by disturbances in the usual flow of energy, i.e. from positive to neutral to negative and back.

Practitioners use their hands and fingers at various prescribed points to 're-polarize' different fields of the body so that energy can again flow normally and restore health.

The techniques

The aim of polarity is to identify the energy imbalance causing dysfunction.

The practitioner will take a detailed medical history including the presenting complaint, past medical history, medication, allergies and lifestyle (smoking, alcohol, exercise). The patient's diet is looked at with emphasis on typical daily intake. The patient's body language in response to certain questions is a particlarly important aid to history taking.

Element checklist: the five elements are listed together with their corresponding functions and organs (some examples are given in Box 3.1). The practitioner goes down the list, ticking off where the patient has an imbalance.

BOX 3.1 Examples of functions and organs associated with the five elements

Ether	hearing throat grief	**Water**	taste feet balanced	**Earth**	smell neck strong
Air	touch ankles greed	**Fire**	sight head anger		

Patients are asked to remove all metallic objects and jewellery to stop interference with their own energy field. Practitioners will often use a wooden couch for the same reason. Pulse and blood pressure are measured.

Short leg side: the patient lies on the couch. The shorter leg indicates the side of the body with 'contracted' electromagnetic energies.

The respiratory system is examined to check respiratory rate and quality of breathing – a measure of how much *prana* the patient is drawing from the atmosphere. The symmetry and alignment of the body is checked, together with hot and cold areas of skin and the state of the toes and fingers. The latter are useful indicators of energy disturbance. Capillary return in the nails after squeezing is believed to be a direct indication of the flow of *prana*.

Other methods of assessing the state of a patient's energy include pulse diagnosis, hand scanning (moving the hand over the body but making no contact with the skin), dowsing with a pendulum and aura analysis. Once the energy disturbance has been identified the practitioner works with the patient to redress the balance by:

manipulation and massage
exercises, e.g. yoga
relaxation techniques, e.g. meditation
dietary manipulation
herbal or naturopathic treatments.

WHICH CONDITIONS ARE SUITABLE FOR TREATMENT BY POLARITY THERAPY?

- Pain relief:
  - migraine and chronic headaches
  - backache
  - frozen shoulder
  - carpal tunnel syndrome
  - arthritis (rheumatoid, osteoarthritis)
  - gout
  - repetitive strain injury
  - sports injury (see also below)
  - toothache
  - neuralgia
  - other chronic or terminal illnesses

- Psychological:
  - anxiety
  - stress
  - insomnia
  - feeling 'run down'
  - phobias

- Neurological:
  - vertigo

- Allergies:
  - asthma
  - eczema
  - sinus and catarrhal problems
  - urticaria

- Skin:
  - pruritus
  - excessive sweating
  - psoriasis

- Abdominal:
  - peptic ulcer
  - colitis
  - irritable bowel syndrome
  - constipation
  - diverticulitis
  - gallstones
  - haemorrhoids

- Eating disorders:
  - compulsive eating
  - bulimia
  - anorexia

- Addictions:
  smoking
  drugs (including benzodiazepines)
  alcohol

- Urinary:
  kidney stones
  water retention
  cystitis

- Pregnancy:
  labour pain

- Gynaecological:
  premenstrual tension
  menopausal symptoms
  candidiasis (thrush)
  painful, heavy, irregular periods

- Metabolic:
  non-insulin dependent diabetes
  hyperlipidaemia (high cholesterol level)
  obesity

- Post-viral fatigue syndrome

- Convalescence

WHICH CONDITIONS ARE NOT SUITABLE FOR TREATMENT BY POLARITY THERAPY?

- Any illness that may be caused by serious underlying disease
- Serious infections
- Inflammation or infection of veins or lymphatics
- Deep vein thrombosis
- Shingles
- Scar tissue
- Varicose veins
- Serious psychiatric illness
- Epilepsy

Advantages

- Safe.
- Very few side-effects.
- Does not interact with patient's existing medication.

Disadvantages

- Deep massage can be painful.
- Occasional healing crisis with aggravation of symptoms as toxins are released.
- Cost borne by the patient.
- Practitioners not easily available.

How long and how much?

First session: 1 hour.
Subsequent sessions: 30 minutes to 1 hour.
How many sessions? Up to six recommended.
Cost: £20–30 (1996 UK prices).

NHS or private? (applicable to the UK only)

Polarity therapy is not available on the NHS.

Addresses for referral

British Complementary Medicine
Association
9 Soar Lane
Leicester LE3 5DE
Tel. 01162 425406

UK Polarity Therapy Association
Monomark House
27 Old Gloucester Street
London WC1N 3XX
Tel. 01483 417714

**Addresses for education
and training**

British Complementary Medicine
Association
(Address above)

International School of Polarity
Therapists
7 Nunney Close
Golden Valley
Cheltenham
Glos GL51 0TU
Tel. 01242 522352

International School of Polarity
Therapy
12–14 Dowell Street
Honiton
Devon EX14 8LT
Tel. 01404 44330

Polarity Therapy Center of San
Francisco
409-A Lawton Street
San Francisco, CA 94122
USA
Tel. 415 753 1298

Rosen method

Background

The Rosen method of bodywork uses a combination of psychotherapy, massage, relaxation and breathing exercises to help clients.
It was first developed by Marion Rosen, a German physiotherapist,
who eventually took her work to Sweden and the USA after the
Second World War.

The key concept of therapy is 'armouring'. Over time, uncomfortable internal psychological and emotional states (fear, embarrass-
ment, anger, etc.) are stored as chronic muscular tension. This is
reflected in the patient's posture and stance.

Reichian therapy or *bioenergetics* has an almost identical techni-
cal approach to the Rosen method. However, as well as armouring,
therapists also believe in a vital life force *chi* (or *prana*) which needs
to be re-balanced to effect therapy. Re-balancing is commonly
achieved by breath control exercises. Interestingly William Reich,
the founder of Reichian therapy, died in prison in 1957 in the
USA. He was convicted as a fraudster by medical contemporaries.
Since his death his theories of armouring and bioenergy have been
highly influential in psychotherapy and related disciplines.

Research

No controlled studies have been carried out on these therapies.

Mechanism of action

The body armour built up from years of uncomfortable psychological and emotional exposure is slowly dismantled by relaxing
muscular tension. This 'armour disrobing' allows patients to recognize their true selves.

The techniques

The practitioner takes a brief history of the ailment, if one is
present. Many healthy clients view it as an exploration into the
self. Through a system of exercises (e.g. maintaining certain postures), light massage and touch, breath control and relaxation, individual muscles begin to relax.

Therapy is often carried out in groups. However, one-to-one
therapy helps the patient focus on breathing and which muscles

to relax. As muscles relax, patients undergo a cathartic process as psychological and emotional memories are released from the body and eventually disappear. Often intense physical reactions such as weeping or shouting are discharged. The presence and psychotherapeutic skills of the therapist give 'permission' to the patient to analyse and gain insight into repressed memories.

As sessions progress, the patient should begin to notice changes in posture, mood and general health.

WHICH CONDITIONS ARE SUITABLE FOR TREATMENT BY THE ROSEN METHOD?

- Musculoskeletal: back pain
                       neck pain
                       arthritis
                       aching joints
                       muscle stiffness
                       cramps

- Minor sports injuries: soft tissue injuries

- Psychological: anxiety
                       stress
                       insomnia
                       depression
                       feeling 'run down'

- Gynaecological: premenstrual tension

- Headaches

- Post-viral fatigue syndrome

- Restless legs

- Jet-lag

- Irritable bowel syndrome

- Progressive conditions: multiple sclerosis
                          Parkinson's disease

- Terminal disease: cancers

WHICH CONDITIONS ARE NOT SUITABLE FOR TREATMENT BY THE ROSEN METHOD?

- Any condition that may be caused by serious underlying disease
- Early pregnancy (before 3 months)
- Sexually transmitted diseases
- Serious infectious disease
- Inflammation or infection of veins or lymphatics
- Deep vein thrombosis
- Shingles
- Scar tissue
- Varicose veins
- Serious psychiatric illness, e.g. schizophrenia

Advantages

- Non-invasive.
- Safe.
- Patients can often experience positive emotional changes.
- Very little equipment is needed.

Disadvantages

- Very difficult to find practitioners in the UK for the Rosen method and Reichian therapy.
- Time and cost may be prohibitive for some.
- Tiredness is a common side-effect.

How long and how much?

First session: 1 hour.
Subsequent sessions: 45–90 minutes.
How many sessions? Ideally weekly or fortnightly. The patient should stop when no further benefits are obvious.
Cost: £35–70 per session (1996 UK prices).

NHS or private? (applicable to the UK only)

These therapies are not available on the NHS.

Addresses for referral

Bioenergetic Partnership
22 Fitzjohn's Avenue
London NW3 5NB
Tel. 0171 435 1079

Institute of Bioenergetic Medicine
103 North Road
Parkstone
Poole
Dorset BH14 0LU
Tel. 01202 733762

Addresses for education and training

Bioenergetic Partnership
(see above)
(Foundation course, one Saturday every
month for a year)

The 3-year course for a Rosen method
practitioner is only available from the
USA or Scandinavia.

4

Oral therapies

Homoeopathy

Background

The basics of homoeopathy were discovered by Dr Samuel Hahnemann, a prominent German doctor in the late eighteenth century. It was during an epidemic of swamp fever that he discovered that cinchona bark, the standard treatment for the condition at the time, actually gave symptoms of swamp fever if taken in high enough doses. Hahnemann and his colleagues experimented further with many other substances to observe their action on healthy individuals. This process was called 'proving'. When sick people were treated with the resulting 'remedies' it was found that some of their symptoms actually became worse. Dilution of the original dosage often produced a cure without side-effects. Hahnemann discovered that violent shaking or 'succussion' during dilution increased potency while rendering the substance less toxic. This process of 'like cures like' was explained by Hahnemann in terms of the presence of a 'vital force' in every substance helping to re-energize the vital force in the sick individual, so effecting cure.

Hahnemann's ideas of the fundamental causes of disease were also non-conventional. He believed that ill-health was caused by two flaws in the constitution. First, residues of old illnesses (toxins or infections) and deep-seated genetic predispositions could affect an individual's state of health. He called these susceptibilities 'miasms'. Second, defective or depleted cellular function (caused by physical or psychological stress) could leave the body open to further illness and susceptible to the long-term effects of miasms. This constitutional state was called 'psora'.

Modern homoeopathy now covers about 2000 remedies (plant, mineral and occasionally animal) which are described in the standard text *Materia Medica*. Many practitioners also use the

Repertory, an encyclopaedia of symptoms (arranged in systems such as Mind, Head, Eyes, etc.) with a list of suitable remedies. Using this guide, which is now available in the form of computer software, the practitioner is able to choose the most appropriate remedy.

Research

Homoeopathy is one of the few fields of complementary medicine in which serious research has been done and come out in its favour.

- Reilly, D. T., Taylor, M. A., Beattie, G. *et al.* (1986). Is homoeopathy a placebo response? Controlled trial of homoeopathic potency with pollen in hayfever as a model. *The Lancet*, **2**(8512): 881–6.

This double-blind crossover study on hay fever showed a statistical superiority of homoeopathic treatment to placebo.

- Fisher, P., Greenwood, A., Huskisson, E. C. *et al.* (1989). Effect of homoeopathic treatment on fibrositis (primary fibromyalgia). *British Medical Journal*, **299**: 365–6.

A study on fibromyalgia indicated that varying dilutions or 'potencies' of homoeopathic substances did exert measurable effects.

- Klijnen, J., Knipschild, P., ter Riet, G. (1991). Clinical trials of homoeopathy. *British Medical Journal*, **302**(6772): 316–23.

This met-analysis study of homoeopathic trials indicated that out of 105 trials, 81 gave positive results in favour of homoeopathy compared to placebo.

- Reilly, D. T., Taylor, M. A., Beattie, G. *et al.* (1994). Is evidence for homoeopathy reproducible? *The Lancet*, **344**(8937): 1601–6.

In this study, 28 patients with allergic asthma were randomly allocated to receive either a homoeopathic remedy or placebo. A significant difference in therapies appeared within 1 week of starting therapy and persisted for 8 weeks.

Recently some parents have become keen on the idea of homoeopathy as an alternative to childhood immunization. There is no evidence whatsoever that homoeopathic vaccines work. The Council of the Faculty of Homoeopathy (medically qualified homoeopaths) supports conventional immunization. The Society of Homoeopaths (non-medically qualified practitioners) opposes immunization.

Mechanism of action

Much scepticism still surrounds homoeopathy with its two main tenets of 'like cures like' and 'less is more' (dilution). Homoeopathic protagonists will often, however, give the example of modern 'attenuated' vaccines. These are viruses so highly diluted that they do not cause disease but do stimulate the body's defences. Some of the theories put forward to explain the effects of homoeopathy can be summarized as follows:

● Remedies stimulate the body into repairing itself.
● The body is extremely sensitive to the homoeopathic remedy needed to effect cure, as illustrated by the high dilutions used – many well in excess of one part per million.
● High dilution or 'high potency' remedies may act on energy flow in the body and not on physical processes.
● Succussion or shaking the remedy during dilution potentiates its effects by leaving an 'imprint' of the remedy in the solution – perhaps homoeopathic substances are involved not in chemical processes but merely in the transmission of information at a molecular level.

The techniques

After taking a detailed history of the patient's problem the homoeopath will go on to analyse the patient's general health and constitution. A detailed analysis is required because the patient is treated as a whole. Patients with the same problem may well require different remedies. The investigation will cover the patient's family and social history, preference of temperatures, favourite types of food, personality, sleep patterns, and allergies.

When the therapist has built up a detailed picture of the malady *and* the patient, a remedy can be chosen. For simple problems like bruising, hay fever and soft-tissue injuries the remedy is straightforward. For anything more complex the *Materia Medica* or *Repertory* are referred to.

Remedies are often available over the counter from chemists or a homoeopathic pharmacist. General practitioners who practise homoeopathy are able to write the prescription on their usual prescription pads (form FP10).

Dilution (or potency) of the remedies is varied according to the malady being treated. The homoeopath may start off with a lower potency, e.g. 6C (i.e. a dilution of 1×10^6), and work up to 30C (a *higher* dilution of 1×10^{30}). Some remedies can go up to dilutions of 10M (1×1000^{10}).

Many homoeopaths will prepare the remedy at their practice. A calculated number of drops of the remedy are added to a quantity of sugar pills. The pills containing the absorbed medicine are then taken as directed. Occasionally drops or a liquid preparation will be dispensed. The effects of homoeopathic remedies are thought to be increased by absorption through the lining of the mouth.

- Precaution with the pills:
    avoid exposure to sunlight
    avoid exposure to strong smells
    avoid touching the pills, sweat renders them ineffective
    the pills should be *sucked* not swallowed
    do not take anything by mouth 20 minutes before or after a pill (even toothpaste or drinks)
    the pills can be degraded by X-rays (avoid passing through security machines).
- Drops or liquids should be held in the mouth for 10 seconds before swallowing.
- One remedy is usually given at a time. The homoeopath will review the patient after a course of pills. If the patient is no better the therapist may question the patient again and try a different potency or remedy.

Side-effects
Symptoms may rarely worsen – a good sign usually but often means that the body is being overstimulated. Stop taking the pills for one week or until the symptoms settle, then re-start.

Homoeopathic podiatry
Homoeopathic treatment is becoming increasingly popular for difficult nail and foot problems. Topical homoeopathic and 'marigold therapy' treatments are applied together with orthodox chiropody.

WHICH CONDITIONS ARE SUITABLE FOR HOMOEOPATHIC TREATMENT?

- Pain relief:

  migraine and chronic headaches
  backache
  frozen shoulder
  carpal tunnel syndrome
  arthritis (rheumatoid, osteoarthritis)
  gout
  repetitive strain injury
  sports injury (see also below)
  toothache
  neuralgia
  other chronic or terminal illnesses

- Psychological:

  anxiety
  stress
  insomnia
  feeling 'run down'
  phobias

- Neurological:

  Bell's palsy
  vertigo
  Ménière's disease

- Allergies:

  asthma
  hay fever
  eczema
  sinus and catarrhal problems
  urticaria

- Skin:

  mouth ulcers
  chronic leg ulcers
  pruritus
  excessive sweating
  acne
  psoriasis

- Abdominal:

  peptic ulcer
  colitis
  irritable bowel syndrome
  constipation
  diverticulitis
  gallstones
  haemorrhoids
  worms

- Eating disorders: compulsive eating
                           bulimia
                           anorexia

- Addictions: smoking
                           drugs (including benzodiazepines)
                           alcohol

- Urinary: Bed-wetting in children
                           kidney stones
                           water retention
                           cystitis

- Pregnancy: nausea and vomiting
                           labour pain

- Gynaecological: premenstrual tension
                           menopausal symptoms
                           candidiasis (thrush)
                           painful, heavy, irregular periods

- Metabolic: non-insulin dependent diabetes
                           hyperlipidaemia (high cholesterol level)
                           obesity

- Mouth problems: halitosis
                           stomatitis
                           ulcers
                           candidiasis (thrush)

- Children: hyperactivity/behavioural problems
                           nappy rash
                           sleep problems
                           teething
                           colic

- Injuries and accidents: bites and stings
                           bruises
                           burns and scalds
                           sprains and strains
                           sunburn
                           travel sickness

- Foot problems: corns
                           calluses
                           bunions
                           inflamed joints
                           chilblains
                           dry eczema
                           athlete's foot
                           ulcers

- Twitchy eyes
- Nausea and vomiting from anaesthesia or motion
- Tinnitus
- Ear wax
- Post-viral fatigue syndrome
- Convalescence

WHICH CONDITIONS ARE NOT SUITABLE FOR HOMOEOPATHIC TREATMENT?

- Any condition that may be caused by serious underlying disease
- Serious infections
- Epilepsy
- Serious musculoskeletal injury
- Terminal illness (e.g. cancer)

Homoeopathy may be used as an *adjunct* to conventional therapy in serious injuries or terminal disease.

Note: Vegetarians should be aware that some remedies are animal-based, e.g. sepia (cuttlefish ink), lachesis (snake venom) and apis (bees).

Advantages

- Safe (even in early pregnancy and in children).
- Very few side-effects.
- Does not interact with patient's existing medication.
- Popular with the general public.
- Economical; most remedies are much cheaper than conventional drugs.
- GPs are able to write medication on the usual prescription pad.

Disadvantages

- 'Externalization' of the disease may produce skin changes (rashes, boils), diarrhoea or catarrh. This often indicates that the body is starting to heal itself.

- Not usually available on the NHS unless the patient's own GP is a homoeopath.
- Cost is borne by the patient.
- Homoeopathic consultations often take much longer than orthodox consultations.
- 'Less is more' concept difficult to accept by orthodox doctors.

How long and how much?

First appointment: up to 1 hour.
Subsequent appointments: 30 minutes to 1 hour.
How many sessions? Occasionally only one is required. Some patients may need up to six sessions.
Cost: £70–90 for first session; subsequent sessions are £35–50 *plus* cost of remedy (1996 UK prices).

NHS or private? (applicable to the UK only)

- **NHS:** not usually available on the NHS. However, some general practitioners are able to refer their patients to the Royal London Homoeopathic Hospital for NHS treatment.
- **Private:** widely available privately. An increasing number of doctors are also practising homoeopathy. Refer only to members of the relevant professional organization.

Simple self-help measures

These self-help measures are all available from local or homoeopathic pharmacists. If problems persist or worsen a doctor should be consulted.

Children

- Teething:
    chamomilla granules.
- Nappy rash:
    calendula cream.
- Colds:
    aconite – take at onset
    natrium muriaticum (nat. mur.) – sneezing
    mercurius solubilis (merc. sol.) – feverish head cold.
- Sore throat:
    arsenicum album (arsen alb.) – dry, burning
    bryonia – soothes.

- Indigestion:
  carbo vegetabilis (carbo veg.) – wind
  kalium phosphoricum (kali. phos.).
- Colic:
  colocynth
  magnesium phosphoricum (mag. phos.).

Gynaecological problems

- Painful periods:
  belladonna
  pulsatilla.
- Menopausal symptoms:
  pulsatilla
  sepia.
- Premenstrual tension:
  nat. mur. – mood swings
  pulsatilla
  sepia – colic or upset stomach.
- Cystitis:
  belladonna – burning
  cantharis – burning
  pulsatilla – urgency to pass water.

Pregnancy

- Nausea and vomiting:
  ipecac
  nux vomica.

Minor injuries

- Pain, bruising:
  arnica cream
  hypericum cream – broken skin, sensitive areas, e.g. fingers or toes
  ruta graveolens (ruta grav.).

Gastrointestinal problems

- Irritable bowel syndrome:
  colocynth
  mag. phos.

Addresses for referral

British Homoeopathic Association
27a Devonshire Street
London WC1N 1RJ
Tel. 0171 935 2163

Faculty of Homoeopathy
Royal London Homoeopathic Hospital
Great Ormond Street
London WC1N 3HR
Tel. 0171 837 3091

Homoeopathic Hospital
1000 Great Western Road
Glasgow G12 0NR
Tel. 0141 339 0382

Homoeopathic Trust Faculty of
Homoeopathy
Hahnemann House
2 Powis Place
London WC1N 3HT
Tel. 0171 837 9469

National Center for Homoeopathy
801 North Fairfax Street
Alexandria, VA 22314
USA
Tel. 703 548 7790

Society of Homoeopaths
2 Artisan Road
Northampton NN1 4HU
Tel. 01604 21400

Addresses for education and training

Homoeopathic Hospital, Glasgow
(Address above; trains doctors only)

Royal London Homoeopathic Hospital
(Address above; trains doctors only)

School of Homoeopathic Medicine
46 Long Meadow Road
Alfreton
Derbyshire EE5 7PD
Tel. 01773 831291

Scottish College of Homoeopathy
17 Queens Crescent
Glasgow G4 9BL
Tel. 0141 332 3917

Herbal medicine

Background

The use of plant materials to maintain health and treat illness goes back to the earliest civilizations. The first practitioners probably prescribed herbs according to taste, texture, colour and their immediate effect. Over centuries of trial and error a system of therapeutics evolved and was disseminated throughout the world by travellers, trade and invasion. The first known records date back to the Chinese and Egyptians, around 2500 BC. Many of these teachings were then taken up and formalized by Greek, Roman and Islamic healers. From the Moghuls in Turkey and Spain, the art of herbalism spread to the rest of Europe in the sixteenth and seventeenth centuries and from there it was a natural progression to North America a hundred years later. Each culture would add new plants and therapies to its own basic system of herbalism while passing on its own ideas and treatments.

Modern herbalism is probably the most commonly practised form of medicine worldwide – almost every village and small town in Asia will have a practitioner or *hakim*; African villagers, and native Americans in both North and South America all practise forms of herbal medicine; orthodox practitioners in China practise allopathic and herbal medicine side by side. An increasing number of medical practitioners in the West are discovering the benefits of herbal medicine and are incorporating it into their armoury of treatment. Western pharmaceutical companies and their research pharmacists have always been interested in naturally occurring medicines. This interest is, however, usually coupled with modern therapeutic theories which encourage the identification of the active ingredient. This is then synthesized artificially and made into a saleable product with a precise dosage range.

Herbal pharmacists have a different point of view. They argue that the substances present in their herbal concoctions arc naturally well balanced which helps to neutralize their unwanted actions. This, together with weak dilutions, keeps the incidence of side-effects to a minimum.

Traditional Chinese herbalism
Traditional Chinese herbalism differs from Western herbal medicine mainly in its philosophy. Chinese herbalism is the fourth part of traditional Chinese medicine (TCM). Acupuncture, food cures and manipulation are its three other components. The rebalancing of *yin* and *yang* and in turn the circulation of *chi* (internal energy) is the main strategy of TCM. Thus herbs are classified according to their effects on this energy flow, i.e. do they cool, heat, dry or moisten *chi*. Although Chinese herbalism also uses mineral and animal products, many of the herbal remedies used are the same as in Western herbalism.

Research

Despite the long history and popularity of herbal medicine, comparatively little research work has been done on its efficacy. There are over half a million plants on Earth – only 5% have been through the hands of researchers. Fortunately, with interest increasing amongst the general population, research also appears to be attracting attention. Regular studies are coming out of India,

70   Complementary Medicine: a practical guide

Japan and China, and the Hamdard Institute, Karachi, Pakistan, and the World Health Organization (WHO) are evaluating traditional herbal remedies for use by all. The National Cancer Institute in the USA has appraised over 20 000 plant species for use as antitumour agents.

Many countries have active programmes to safeguard plants traditionally used for herbal medicine.

Summary of worldwide research findings

- **Garlic** is antibacterial and antifungal, and helps reduce cholesterol levels (see 'Nutrition' section).
- **Ginger** helps nausea and vomiting, motion sickness, morning sickness.
- **Liquorice root** is useful in healing stomach ulcers.
- **Onion** helps reduce cholesterol levels.
- **Thyme** is antibacterial.
- **Aloe vera** helps wound healing, improves blood circulation, and is anti-inflammatory, antibacterial and antifungal (see 'Aloe vera' section).
- **Capsicum cream** (chili peppers) reduces pain and tenderness in arthritic joints.
- **Valerian root** is anxiolytic and induces sleep.
- **Cranberry juice** reduces painful urination in cystitis, helps reduce stickiness of bacteria (*Escherichia coli*) to the bladder wall.
- **Evening primrose oil** reduces breast pain, and relieves itch and severity in eczema.

The 'standardized teabag study' of eczema was carried out at The Hospital for Sick Children at Great Ormond Street, London, in 1991; the active ingredient was Chinese herbs. More than 60% of the patients aged between 18 months and 18 years saw a marked improvement in their condition. The researchers are planning another trial to test individual mixtures against the standardized 'teabag', based on the premise of herbal medicine that each patient is prescribed a different herbal concoction.

Mechanism of action

Current theories include the following.

Herbs support the 'vital force' present in all living creatures to help maintain health and effect cure.

Herbal medicines elicit a protective physiological response from the body. A side-effect of this response is an improvement of the ailment.

The herb acts as a food to supply the tissues with vital nutrients needed to regain normal cellular function.

Herbs increase the detoxification of the body by enhancing the action of the organs of excretion – liver, kidneys, bowels, sweat glands and lungs.

The techniques

A herbal consultation involves a full medical history including the nature and history of the present complaint, past medical history, medication, emotional functions and family history. In addition a detailed social history is taken including occupation, exercise and eating habits. As in homoeopathy, the practitioner will seek to define the person as a whole.

A physical examination may also be carried out including blood pressure, palpation of the physiological systems (respiratory, cardiovascular, gastrointestinal, etc.) and microscopic analysis of the urine. A Chinese herbalist may also include pulse and tongue diagnosis. Other practitioners may replace the physical examination altogether with other diagnostic methods such as iridology (see Chapter 8).

The main ailment will be treated primarily. Herbs are usually prescribed in combinations of between 2 and 12. The remedy is taken in the form of a pill, powder or tincture (herb extract in alcohol or water). Occasionally the herbs are put into a teabag and the 'tea' is made in the usual way. Over-the-counter treatments are rare and herbalists will usually make up remedies themselves.

Dietary advice is also given. Most patients will be asked to follow a simple, non-refined diet with plenty of fresh fruit and vegetables. Chinese herbalists may give specific instructions, e.g. a patient who has a 'damp' condition such as eczema or asthma should avoid dairy products.

WHICH CONDITIONS ARE SUITABLE FOR HERBAL TREATMENT?

- Pain relief:
  migraine and chronic headaches
  backache
  frozen shoulder
  arthritis (rheumatoid, osteoarthritis)
  gout
  repetitive strain injury
  sports injury (see also below)
  bursitis
  toothache
  neuralgia
  chronic and terminal illnesses

- Psychological:
  anxiety
  stress
  insomnia
  feeling 'run down'

- Neurological:
  Bell's palsy
  Ménière's disease

- Allergies:
  asthma
  hay fever
  eczema
  sinus and catarrhal problems
  urticaria

- Skin:
  mouth ulcers
  chronic leg ulcers
  pruritus
  excessive sweating
  acne
  psoriasis

- Abdominal:
  indigestion
  peptic ulcer
  colitis
  irritable bowel syndrome
  constipation
  diverticulitis
  gallstones
  haemorrhoids
  worms

- Eating disorders:
  compulsive eating
  bulimia
  anorexia

- Addictions: smoking
                             drugs (including benzodiazepines)
                             alcohol

- Urinary: Bed-wetting
                             kidney stones
                             water retention
                             cystitis

- Pregnancy: nausea and vomiting
                             labour pain

- Gynaecological: premenstrual tension
                             menopausal symptoms
                             candidiasis (thrush)
                             menstrual problems

- Metabolic: non-insulin dependent diabetes
                             hyperlipidaemia (high cholesterol level)
                             obesity

- Mouth problems: halitosis
                             stomatitis
                             ulcers
                             candidiasis (thrush)

- Children: hyperactivity and behavioural problems
                             nappy rash
                             sleep problems
                             teething
                             colic
                             colds
                             sore throats
                             indigestion
                             bed-wetting

- Injuries and accidents: bites and stings
                             bruises
                             burns and scalds
                             sprains and strains
                             sunburn
                             travel sickness

- Twitching eyes

- Nausea and vomiting from anaesthesia or motion

- Tinnitus

- Post-viral fatigue syndrome

WHICH CONDITIONS ARE NOT SUITABLE FOR HERBAL TREATMENT?

- Any condition that may be caused by serious underlying disease
- Serious infections
- Serious psychiatric illness, e.g. schizophrenia
- Epilepsy

Advantages

- Safe if prescribed by a professional herbalist (even in pregnant women and in children).
- Few side-effects.
- Few adverse reactions with patient's existing medication.
- Popular with the general public.

Disadvantages

- Adverse effects of some Chinese herbs have resulted in hospital admission for some patients. In the UK, registered Chinese herbalists have supported proposals to control the quality of herbs being imported into the country and to set up a reference laboratory at Kew Gardens.
- Some herbs available over the counter may have unwanted side-effects.
- Healing crisis may occur with aggravation of symptoms. This usually indicates that toxins are being removed from the body.
- Not usually available on the NHS unless the GP is also a herbalist.
- Cost is borne by the patient.
- Doctors are not able to give herbal drugs on prescription.
- Herbal consultations often take much longer than orthodox consultations.

How long and how much?

First appointment: up to 1 hour.
Subsequent appointments: 30 minutes to 1 hour.
How many sessions? Occasionally only one is required. Some patients may need up to six sessions.
Cost: £40–60 per session *plus* cost of herbal remedy (1996 UK prices).

NHS or private? (applicable to the UK only)

- **NHS:** not available on the NHS unless the patient's GP is also a herbalist.
- **Private:** not as widely available as homoeopaths. Refer only to members of professional bodies.

Simple self-help measures

Up to four herbs can be used together; use equal quantities to prepare the remedy. Some suggestions for treatment are given in Box 4.1.

BOX 4.1 Self-help herbal remedies

●	Anaemia	Parsley (add to meals) Nettle tea
●	Colds, sinusitis	Rosemary or marsh-mallow in a bowl of hot water and inhale
●	Cystitis	Yarrow tea Cranberry juice
●	Headache	Rosemary tea Peppermint tea
●	Indigestion	Peppermint tea Fennel tea Chamomile tea
●	Sore throat	Fennel gargle Red sage gargle
●	Vaginal infection	Calendula/marigold soaks

Teas and infusions
For leaves and flowers, use 1 teaspoon per cup of boiling water; cover and leave to infuse for 5–10 minutes.

For roots and bark, boil 1 teaspoon per cup in water for 10–15 minutes.

Strain the tea, and add honey if desired. *Never* add milk or sugar.

Baths
Prepare the herbs as for tea. Add the liquid to bath water and soak.

Addresses for referral

American Herbalists Guild
Box 1683
Soquel, CA 95073
USA
Tel. 408 438 1700

Chi Clinic
6th Floor
Riverbank House
Putney Bridge Approach
Putney
London SW6 3JD
Tel. 0171 222 1888
(Traditional Chinese herbalism)

National Institute of Medical Herbalists
56 Longbrook Street
Exeter EX4 6AH
Tel. 01392 426022

Addresses for education and training

International College of Oriental
Medicine
Green Hedges House
Green Hedges Avenue
East Grinstead
Sussex RH19 1DZ
Tel. 01342 313106/7

London School of Acupuncture and
Traditional Chinese Medicine
3rd Floor
36 Featherstone Street
London EC1Y 6QX
Tel. 0171 490 0513

School of Phytotherapy
Bucksteep Manor
Bodle Street Green
Hailsham
East Sussex BN27 4RJ
Tel. 01323 833812

Bach flower remedies

Background

In 1930 Dr Edward Bach, after many years as a successful physician and homoeopath in England, gave up his practice to study further the relationship between physical disease, personality and emotional imbalance. Bach believed different emotions (fears, worry, anxiety, etc.) could significantly affect the self-healing properties of the body. Different personalities would be affected in different ways.

Bach developed his new system of therapy in Wales, where he examined the effect of plant essences on different moods and emotions. He classified personality disturbance into seven distinct types, characterized by loneliness, fear, indecision, despondency or despair, overcare for the welfare of others, insufficient interest and oversensitivity. These were then subdivided into 38 'states of mind' for which Bach collected 38 flower remedies – each one helping to counter a particular state of mind and the sorts of emotions that people face every day.

The flower remedies are prepared in two different ways. The 'sun' method involves steeping petals in water and exposing to sunlight for 3 hours. The 'heat' method involves boiling the flowers for 30 minutes. In each case brandy is added to the filtered water to make a 'mother tincture'. The latter is then heavily diluted in a grape alcohol solution to form the saleable product.

Rescue Remedy is probably the most famous of the Bach flower remedies. It is a combination of five other remedies (cherry plum, impatiens, rock rose, clematis and star of Bethlehem) and is recommended for stress, emotional or physical trauma and minor bruising.

Research

No controlled studies have been done to study the effects of Bach flower remedies.

Mechanism of action

Water becomes 'potentized' with the healing properties of the flower on exposure to sunlight or boiling. Compare this with the potentization of homoeopathic remedies by succussion.

The techniques

Bach flower remedies are primarily self-help medicines although many complementary practitioners combine them with their own therapies. The remedies are available over the counter in most countries (except Germany where they are prescription medicines), in a 10-ml or 20-ml bottle with a dropper. Self-help books can be used as a simple guide for use in the home.

- How to take the remedy:
    2–3 drops on the tongue every 3–4 hours
    add 2–3 drops to water or juice and sip slowly
    rub on lips, wrist, temples, behind ears
    add a few drops to water and use as a compress in minor injuries
- Rescue Remedy is also available as a cream, for bruising.

WHICH CONDITIONS ARE SUITABLE FOR TREATMENT WITH BACH FLOWER REMEDIES?

- Pain relief: migraine and other headaches
- Psychological: anxiety
                         stress
                         insomnia
                         feeling 'run down'
                         phobias
- Allergies: asthma
- Gastrointestinal: nausea
- Eating disorders: bulimia
                         anorexia
- Addictions: smoking
                         drugs
                         alcohol
- Gynaecological: menopausal problems
                         menstrual problems
                         premenstrual tension
- Pregnancy: nausea and vomiting
                         labour pain
- Metabolic: obesity
- Children's problems: anxiety
                         behavioural problems
                         hyperactivity
                         insomnia
                         bed-wetting
- Minor injuries: bruising
                         faints
                         minor burns

WHICH CONDITIONS ARE NOT SUITABLE FOR TREATMENT WITH BACH FLOWER REMEDIES?

- Any condition that may be caused by serious underlying disease
- Serious infections
- Serious psychiatric illness, e.g. schizophrenia
- Epilepsy

Advantages

- Very safe, even in pregnancy and for children.
- Very few side-effects.
- Simple to use at home.
- Remedies can be used to treat animals.
- Remedies widely available at pharmacies and health-food shops.

Disadvantages

- Remedies can be expensive.
- Not suitable for teetotallers (alcohol content of remedy).

How long and how much?

Remedies are available over the counter. Length of treatment will vary for each individual, depending on symptoms and personality. Chronic problems may need months of therapy.
Typical costs: £2.75 for 10 ml; Rescue Remedy drops £4.50; Rescue Remedy cream £3.30 (1996 UK prices).

NHS or private? (applicable to the UK only)

Bach flower remedies are not available on the NHS.

Simple self-help measures

- Rescue Remedy:
    stress, physical, mental or emotional trauma, a distressed child
    Rescue Remedy cream is used for bruising.
- Olive:
    lethargy, feeling 'run down'.
- Crab apple:
    add to water and use to cleanse boils, spots or infected bites.
- Aspen:
    apprehension, anxiety.

Addresses for referral

Many complementary practitioners use Bach flower remedies regularly in their practice. See under specific therapies.

**Addresses for education
and training**

Bach Flower Centre
Mount Vernon
Bauers Lane
Brightwell cum Stotwell
Wallingford
Oxfordshire OX10 0PZ
Tel. 01491 834678

The Healing Herbs of Dr Bach
PO Box 65
Hereford
HR2 0UW
Tel. 01873 890218

Ayurveda

Background

Ayurveda, the Indian philosophy of medicine, dates back to beyond 2000 BC. Ancient Hindu writings (*Vedas*) indicate that practitioners had great insight into human function and the treatment of ailments. They used basic diagnostic tools (e.g. proctoscopes), carried out suturing after surgery, conceived the idea of microscopic pathogenic organisms and had access to thousands of herbal remedies.

Like Chinese medicine, ayurvedic treatment is based on realigning internal and external energy or *prana* to promote continued health and effect cure.

Unani-tibb developed as a combination of ayurveda and Arabic medicine and is now mainly practised in Pakistan and neighbouring parts of India.

Siddha medicine, another branch of ayurveda which tends to use more minerals, is largely seen in Sri Lanka and southern India.

Research

The vast majority of research has been done in India and is published in Indian national medical journals. The Hamdard Institute, Karachi, Pakistan and the WHO are researching the effectiveness of Unani-tibb medicine and herbal remedies.

Despite the absence of convincing double-blind crossover studies, the usefulness and popularity of ayurveda and its related practices appears to be increasingly recognized in the West.

Mechanism of action

Practitioners believe that disease is caused by an imbalance between the body's natural energies. These are called *doshas*. There are three types:

Vata controls musculoskeletal and nervous systems.
Pitta controls biochemistry and digestion.
Kapha controls cell and tissue growth.

Therapy aims to re-balance this energy disturbance.

A further theory is that ayurvedic medicines elicit a protective physiological response from the body. A side-effect of this response is an improvement of the ailment.

Herbs also act as a food to supply the tissues with vital nutrients needed to regain normal cellular function.

Ayurvedic medicines are thought to increase the detoxification of the body by enhancing the action of the organs of excretion (liver, kidneys, bowels, sweat glands and lungs).

The techniques

A full medical history, including nature and history of the ailment, past medical history, medication, allergies, family history and social history (smoking, alcohol, occupation), sleep patterns, diet and personality, is taken before treatment is instigated. This is followed by a physical examination, including the chest, abdomen, eyes and voice, and detailed examination of the urine and sweat.

Practitioners use various additional techniques for diagnosis:

date of birth and 'astrological diagnosis'
palmistry
pulse and tongue diagnosis.

As in homoeopathy and herbal medicine the practitioner will formulate a remedy to suit the individuality of that patient. Remedies are in a powder form or a tincture. Dietary advice, yoga, breathing exercises, massage, sweat baths, purgatives, enemas and nasal cleaning may also be recommended.

Some practitioners may treat patients with *chavutti thirumal* – a special form of Indian massage using the feet to rub down the body.

WHICH CONDITIONS ARE SUITABLE FOR AYURVEDIC TREATMENT?

- Pain relief:
  - migraine and chronic headaches
  - backache
  - frozen shoulder
  - arthritis (rheumatoid, osteoarthritis)
  - gout
  - repetitive strain injury
  - sports injury (see also below)
  - bursitis
  - toothache
  - neuralgia
  - chronic and terminal illnesses

- Psychological
  - anxiety
  - stress
  - insomnia
  - feeling 'run down'

- Neurological:
  - Bell's palsy
  - Ménière's disease

- Allergies:
  - asthma
  - hay fever
  - eczema
  - sinus and catarrhal problems
  - urticaria

- Skin:
  - mouth ulcers
  - chronic leg ulcers
  - pruritus
  - excessive sweating
  - acne
  - psoriasis

- Abdominal:
  - indigestion
  - peptic ulcer
  - colitis
  - irritable bowel syndrome
  - constipation
  - diverticulitis
  - gallstones
  - haemorrhoids
  - worms

- Eating disorders:
  - compulsive eating
  - bulimia
  - anorexia

- Addictions: smoking
                          drugs (including benzodiazepines)
                          alcohol

- Urinary: Bed-wetting
                          kidney stones
                          water retention
                          cystitis

- Gynaecological: premenstrual tension
                          menopausal symptoms
                          candidiasis (thrush)
                          menstrual problems

- Metabolic: non-insulin dependent diabetes
                          hyperlipidaemia (high cholesterol level)
                          obesity

- Mouth problems: halitosis
                          stomatitis
                          ulcers
                          candidiasis (thrush)

- Children: hyperactivity and behavioural problems
                          nappy rash
                          sleep problems
                          teething
                          colic
                          colds
                          sore throats
                          indigestion
                          bed-wetting

- Injuries and accidents: bites and stings
                          bruises
                          burns and scalds
                          sprains and strains
                          sunburn
                          travel sickness

- Nausea and vomiting from anaesthesia or motion

- Tinnitus

- Post-viral fatigue syndrome

- Tuberculosis

WHICH CONDITIONS ARE NOT SUITABLE FOR AYURVEDIC TREATMENT?

- Any condition that may be caused by serious underlying disease
- Serious infections
- Serious psychiatric illness, e.g. schizophrenia
- Epilepsy

Advantages

- Safe.
- Very few side-effects.
- Does not interact with patient's existing medication.

Disadvantages

- Some traditional ayurvedic medicines may contain mercury or lead – these must be avoided.
- Difficulty in finding a practitioner in the UK. Most work in areas where there is a large immigrant population from the Indian subcontinent. Practitioners are known as '*hakims*' or '*vaids*'.
- No recognized professional body for referral or training in the UK.
- Cost is borne by the patient.

How long and how much?

First appointment: up to 1 hour.
Subsequent appointments: 30 minutes to 1 hour.
How many sessions? Occasionally only one is required. Some patients may need up to six sessions.
Cost: £40 for the first session, £20 for follow-up sessions (1996 UK prices). Cost of the remedy may be extra.

NHS or private? (applicable in the UK only)

Ayurvedic treatment is not available on the NHS.

Simple self-help measures

- Indigestion: 'tea' made from fennel and cardamom.
- High cholesterol levels: increase the amount of chickpeas in the diet.

Addresses for referral

Ayurvedic Centre of Great Britain
50 Penywern Road
London SW5 9SX
Tel. 0171 370 2255

Ayurvedic Living
PO Box 188
Exeter EX4 5AY
(Send A4-size stamped addressed envelope)

Addresses for education and training

American Institute of Vedic Studies
PO Box 8357
Santa Fe, NM 87501
USA
Tel. 505 983 9385
(Correspondence course)

Ayurvedic Centre of Great Britain
(address above)

Ayurvedic Institute and Wellness Centre
PO Box 23445
Albuquerque, NM 87192–1445
USA
Tel. 505 291 9698
(Correspondence course)

Ayurvedic Living
(Address above)

Indian Embassy
Cultural Attaché
India House
Aldwych
London WC2
Tel. 0171 836 8484
(Will provide details of courses in India)

Institute for Wholistic Education
33719 116th Street Box SH
Twin Lakes, WI 53181
USA
Tel. 414 889 8501
(Correspondence course)

Naturopathy

Background

Many practitioners claim that the tenets of naturopathy go back over 4000 years to the time of Hippocrates, who emphasized nature's healing powers and the use of naturally occurring medicines in basic foods. Over the years other treatments as well as dietary manipulation have become incorporated into the art of naturopathy: hydrotherapy (often in spas), fasting, natural hygiene (fresh air, water, sunlight), herbalism, exercise, massage, osteopathy and counselling. Before the industrial revolution the basic ideas of naturopathy (i.e. a sensible diet, exercise and hygiene) had a profound effect on the general population, so much so that these ideas were taken on board by orthodox medical practitioners.

Modernization and urbanization have brought with them their own problems, such as over-refined foods, lack of exercise, occupational illnesses, side-effects from drugs, use of chemicals in farming, and pesticides. No wonder then that an increasingly informed population, especially in the West, is looking at naturopathy and nutritional ideas to counter the effects of such a lifestyle. Many modern naturopaths view themselves as 'natural general practitioners' but, contrary to allopathic medicine, consider that the individual's resistance and ability to overcome disease naturally is paramount. Symptoms of ill-health such as fevers and rashes are seen as signs of the body's vitality and its way of re-establishing health.

Research

Naturopathy in its guise as a multidisciplinary technique has not had any formal research associated with it. Its nutritional branch however, has been the subject of extensive studies (see 'Nutrition' section below).

Mechanism of action

The body tends towards self-regulation or *homoeostasis*. Naturopathy works as a catalyst towards cleansing and detoxifying the body and encouraging self-repairing and self-healing, e.g. a fever will increase the metabolic rate and accelerate blood and lymph circulation, allowing toxins to be eliminated more quickly. Fever also kills bacteria and viruses which thrive at normal body temperature.

Dietary manipulations supply minerals and vitamins essential for maintenance of health and self-healing (see below).

Simple, less refined and organically grown foods contain fewer chemicals than pesticides which can interfere with the body's self-regulatory mechanism.

Drugs prescribed by allopathic practitioners actually interfere with the healing process, often turning an acute illness into a chronic one. Such drugs are eschewed by naturopaths.

Fresh air (e.g. in mountainous areas or near the sea) may be more beneficial because of the presence of large numbers of negative ions. Such ions may work by their lethal effects on bacteria and by reducing plasma levels of histamine (important in allergic conditions such as hay fever or rhinitis).

The techniques

A full medical history is taken including the nature and history of the presenting complaint, past medical history (including fractures and minor ailments), medication, immunizations, allergies, emotional functions and family history. A detailed social history is also taken including smoking and drinking habits, occupation, exercise and food preferences. This is followed by a physical examination including nails, hair and skin. Many naturopaths are also osteopaths and will carefully examine posture, the spinal column and skeletal function.

Other diagnostic tools include chemical analysis of hair (for minerals and toxic metals, e.g. lead and cadmium), blood and urine analysis. Iridology (detailed examination of the iris) is used extensively by naturopaths as a diagnostic aid (see Chapter 8).

Once a diagnosis has been made the practitioner will recommend several changes in lifestyle to help the body cure itself. Naturopaths are mainly non-interventionist. Advice includes dietary measures (fasting, restrictions, supplements), hydrotherapy or spa therapy, exercises, relaxation methods and counselling to encourage a 'positive mental attitude'. Practitioners may also give osteopathic manipulations before the end of the consultation.

Some naturopaths believe that detoxification is the only treatment required and will recommend clay or mud packs, steam baths, mineral baths, etc.

WHICH CONDITIONS ARE SUITABLE FOR NATUROPATHIC TREATMENT?

- Pain relief:
  migraine and chronic headaches
  arthritis (rheumatoid, osteoarthritis)
  gout
  cramp

- Psychological:
  anxiety
  stress
  insomnia
  feeling 'run down'

- Allergies:
  asthma
  hay fever
  eczema
  sinus and catarrhal problems
  urticaria

- Skin: chronic leg ulcers
                               pruritus
                               excessive sweating
                               acne
                               psoriasis

- Abdominal: indigestion
                               peptic ulcer
                               colitis
                               irritable bowel syndrome
                               constipation
                               diverticulitis
                               gallstones
                               haemorrhoids

- Cardiovascular: anaemia
                               blood pressure

- Eating disorders: compulsive eating
                               bulimia
                               anorexia

- Urinary: frequency
                               kidney stones
                               water retention
                               cystitis

- Gynaecological: premenstrual tension
                               menopausal symptoms
                               candidiasis (thrush)
                               menstrual problems

- Metabolic: non-insulin dependent diabetes
                               hyperlipidaemia (high cholesterol level)
                               obesity

- Mouth problems: halitosis
                               candidiasis (thrush)

- Children: hyperactivity and behavioural problems
                               nappy rash
                               sleep problems
                               colic
                               colds
                               indigestion

- Travel sickness
- Nausea and vomiting from anaesthesia or motion
- Post-viral fatigue syndrome
- Hypoglycaemia
- Pregnancy: nausea and vomiting

**WHICH CONDITIONS ARE NOT SUITABLE FOR
NATUROPATHIC TREATMENT?**

- Any condition that may be caused by serious underlying
  disease

- Serious infections

- Serious psychiatric illness, e.g. schizophrenia

- Pain relief for a terminal illness, e.g. cancer

Advantages

- Safe (even in pregnant women and children).
- Very few side-effects.
- Does not interact with the patient's existing medication.
- Increasing in popularity with the general public.
- Holistic – treats the whole patient.

Disadvantages

- Healing crisis can occur as toxins are eliminated from the body.
- Cost is borne by the patient.
- Naturopathic consultations take much longer than orthodox
  consultations.

How long and how much?

First appointment: up to 1 hour.
Subsequent appointments: 30 minutes to 1 hour.
How many sessions? Occasionally only one is required. Some
patients may need regular follow-up sessions.
Cost: £30–50 per session *plus* the cost of supplements (1996 UK
prices).

NHS or private? (applicable to the UK only)

- **NHS:** not available on the NHS.
- **Private:** many practitioners available for referral. Refer only to
  members of professional organizations.

Addresses for referral

American Association of Naturopathic
Physicians
2366 Eastlake Ave East
Seattle, WA 98102
USA
Tel. 206 323 7610

Incorporated Society of British
Naturopaths
The Coach House
293 Gilmerton Road
Edinburgh EH16 5UQ
Tel. 0131 664 3435

General Council and Register of
Naturopaths
Goswell House
2 Goswell Road
Street
Somerset BA16 0JG
Tel. 01458 840072

Address for education
and training

British College of Naturopathy and
Osteopathy
Frazer House
6 Netherhall Gardens
London NW3 5RR
Tel. 0171 435 6464

Nutrition therapy

Background

Nutrition therapy was initially a subdivision of naturopathy but has now developed as a therapy in its own right. Specialists in this field of 'nutritional medicine' began to emerge in the 1950s and started treating disease and promoting health by using supplementary minerals and vitamins together with advice on eliminating toxins and allergens from the diet. Unlike naturopathy with its basic tenets of homoeostasis and self-cure, nutrition therapy is much more interventionist. Practitioners believe that illness comes about as a result of abnormal biochemistry affecting cellular function. Correcting these biochemical aberrations by nutritional manipulation allows the restoration and maintenance of health.

The popularity of nutritional therapy has increased enormously in recent years and has been reflected by an increased demand for less refined foods, organically grown fruit and vegetables and organically reared animals. Orthodox doctors have started to incorporate nutritional advice into their treatment plans for many diseases, e.g. hypertension, diabetes and high cholesterol levels.

In spite of these factors, studies have shown that the general population in 'developed' countries is still eating too much fat and not enough fruit and vegetables. In 1992 the Nutrition Task Force was set up in the UK as a result of the government's *Health of the Nation* White Paper to define what the population should eat to stay healthy. The Task Force published its final report in 1996 and proposed further research into ways of promoting healthy eating, more nutrition classes and cooking skills in schools, and an annual assessment of how things are progressing. The UK's General Medical Council is also realizing the importance of simple nutritional measures and is placing more emphasis on nutrition, health promotion and disease prevention in medical school curricula.

Research

Extensive work has been done on the role of trace elements, minerals and vitamins in human function. In addition, studies have been carried out on certain 'primitive' communities and religious groups to look at the effects of diet on health. The results of some of these studies are attracting the attention of both complementary and orthodox practitioners. For example:

- Vitamin E may have a role in protection from coronary artery disease and cancer (see vitamin E section).
- A study at Edinburgh University found that sufferers with angina had lower plasma levels of vitamin E, vitamin C and beta-carotene.
- The Mediterranean diet which includes salads, lightly cooked vegetables dressed in olive oil, fresh fruit, bread, pasta, rice and plenty of fish and white meat, is being recognized more and more as the best diet to prevent cardiovascular disease.
- Garlic therapy: several studies have indicated that garlic has a number of valuable properties, which include lowering of blood fats, reducing clotting agents (thus reducing thrombosis), thinning the blood and lowering blood pressure (see garlic therapy section).
- Extract from green-lipped mussel (*Perna canaliculus*) may be an effective supplement or alternative to orthodox treatment of rheumatoid arthritis and osteoarthritis (see green-lipped mussel section).
- Vitamin B_6 (pyridoxine) has been found to be effective in premenstrual syndrome.
- Vitamin C and zinc can help wound healing.

- The Inuit (Eskimos) who tend to have a diet very rich in animal fat were found to have a low incidence of heart disease. Further research revealed the presence of high levels of polyunsaturated fats in fish oils, a vital part of the Inuit diet. These findings have led to the development of a drug preparation rich in omega-3 marine triglycerides (Maxepa) which is used in the treatment of raised blood fats.

Mechanism of action

Illness is due to biochemical imbalance. When this is corrected by dietary advice and supplementation, health is restored.

Many problems are caused by allergies or food sensitivities. Exclusion of the allergen or the offending food will effect cure.

Toxic overload may occur owing to chemicals (e.g. pesticides) or heavy metals (e.g. lead) in food or the environment. Build-up of toxins can also occur when the organs of elimination (liver, kidneys, lungs, skin) are affected by disease. Toxins need to be eliminated because they interfere with cellular functions.

Dietary manipulation and supplements correct nutritional deficiencies due to poor diet or malabsorption.

The techniques

A full medical history is taken, including the nature and history of the presenting complaint, past medical history, medication, allergies, personality, family history and details on occupation, smoking and alcohol. A detailed dietary history is essential. Some practitioners will ask the patient to fill in a health questionnaire which serves as a basis for diagnosis. To obtain a detailed analysis of dietary intake, a 'food diary' may need to be kept by the patient for several weeks.

Practitioners will often carry out a full physical examination including nails, hair and skin. Blood and urine may also be analysed. Kinesiology (muscle testing) may be used by some practitioners to elicit food allergens (see Chapter 3).

Once an initial diagnosis has been made the nutritionist may advise a special diet (e.g. hypoallergenic, low fat, high fibre, or cleansing). The diet advised may involve juicing, which allows the nutrients present in fruit and vegetables to be absorbed quickly. Supplements of vitamins, minerals, essential fatty acids and amino acids are also usually prescribed.

Review of the patient after these treatment measures may reveal secondary diagnoses which are treated in the same way.

WHICH CONDITIONS ARE SUITABLE FOR NUTRITIONAL TREATMENT?

- Pain relief:

  migraine and chronic headaches
  arthritis (rheumatoid, osteoarthritis)
  gout
  cramp

- Psychological:

  anxiety
  stress
  insomnia
  feeling 'run down'
  depression

- Allergies:

  asthma
  hay fever
  eczema
  sinus and catarrhal problems
  urticaria

- Skin:

  chronic leg ulcers
  pruritus
  excessive sweating
  acne
  psoriasis

- Abdominal:

  indigestion
  peptic ulcer
  colitis
  irritable bowel syndrome
  constipation
  diverticulitis
  gallstones
  haemorrhoids

- Cardiovascular:

  anaemia
  high blood pressure

- Eating disorders:

  compulsive eating
  bulimia
  anorexia

- Urinary:

  frequency
  kidney stones
  water retention
  cystitis

- Gynaecological: premenstrual tension
                       menopausal symptoms
                       candidiasis (thrush)
                       menstrual problems

- Metabolic: non-insulin dependent diabetes
                       hyperlipidaemia (high cholesterol level)
                       obesity

- Mouth problems: halitosis
                       candidiasis (thrush)

- Children: hyperactivity and behavioural problems
                       nappy rash
                       sleep problems
                       colic
                       colds
                       indigestion

- Travel sickness

- Nausea and vomiting from anaesthesia or motion

- Post-viral fatigue syndrome

- Hypoglycaemia

- Pregnancy: nausea and vomiting

WHICH CONDITIONS ARE NOT SUITABLE FOR NUTRITIONAL TREATMENT?

- Any condition that may be caused by serious underlying disease

- Serious infections

- Serious psychiatric illness, e.g. schizophrenia

- Pain relief for a terminal illness, e.g. cancer

Advantages

- Safe (even in pregnant women and children).
- Very few side-effects.
- Does not interact with patient's existing medication.
- Increasing in popularity with the general public.

Disadvantages

- Cost of consultation *and* supplements may be expensive.
- Consultations take much longer than orthodox consultations.
- Risk of malnutrition from overstrict diets given by inexperienced practitioners.
- Potential dangers of toxic effects of vitamin overdosage – often self-administered by patients.

How long and how much?

First appointment: up to 1 hour.
Subsequent appointments: 30 minutes to 1 hour.
How many sessions? Occasionally only one is required. Some patients may need regular follow-up sessions.
Cost: £30–50 per session *plus* cost of supplements (1996 UK prices).

NHS or private? (applicable to the UK only)

- **NHS:** basic nutrition therapy is available to many NHS patients through dieticians in general practice and hospital. Illnesses particularly treated include diabetes, ischaemic heart disease and gross obesity.
- **Private:** many practitioners available. Refer only to members of professional organizations.

Simple self-help measures

- Digestive problems:
   freshly juiced apples and live goat's yoghurt.
- Detoxification:
   1 day a week on grapes or pears
   3 days on steamed brown rice with steamed vegetables and salad.

Addresses for referral

British Dietetic Association
(Address not available)
Tel. 0121 643 5483
(Patients may need a letter of referral
from their GP before contact)

British Nutrition Foundation
52–54 High Holborn
London WC1V 6RQ
Tel. 0171 404 6504
(Publish *Nutrition Bulletin* and regular
newsletters)

Institute for Optimum Nutrition
Blades Court
Deodar Road
Putney
London SW15 2NU
Tel. 0181 877 9993

Nutritional Eye Health Centre
Sanctuary House
Oulton Road
Oulton
Lowestoft NR32 4QZ
Tel. 01502 583294
(For optical problems)

Addresses for education and training

Centre for Nutritional Studies
Garden House
Rufford Abbey
Newark
Notts NG22 9DE
Tel. 01623 822004

Institute for Optimum Nutrition
(Address above)

Specific nutritional therapies

Aloe vera

Background

Aloe vera (*Aloe barbadensis* Miller) is a member of a genus of succulent herbaceous plants of which there are over 200 species. A stem is usually absent; the fleshy, spiny-toothed leaves form a basal rosette up to half a metre in diameter. The flowers are red or yellow. At first sight aloe vera looks rather like a cactus but is in fact a member of the family Liliaceae (lily) and counts the asparagus, onion and garlic as close relatives. The plant was originally native to Africa but is now grown commercially in favourable climates all over the world.

The aesthetic and medicinal properties of aloe vera appear to have been known for thousands of years with well-documented records from Egyptian, Greek, Indian, Chinese and Roman civilizations. More recently, interest in aloe vera has been rekindled by anecdotal evidence of benefits of treatment in dermatological conditions such as eczema, psoriasis, burns, wounds, ulcers and acne. The scientific community has taken note and an increasing number of studies are being carried out into the properties, constituents and mechanism of action of this plant.

Research

- Davis, R. H., Di Donato, J. J., Johnson, R. W. *et al.* (1994). Aloe vera, hydrocortisone and sterol influence on wound tensile strength and anti-inflammation. *Journal of the American Podiatric Medical Association*, **84**(12): 614–21.

Growth factors in aloe vera mask the wound-healing inhibitors such as sterols and certain amino acids.

- Visuthikosol, V. (1995). Effects of aloe vera gel on healing of burn wounds – a clinical and histologic study. *Journal of the Medical Association of Thailand*, **78**(8): 403–9.

Twenty-seven patients with partial thickness burn wounds were treated with either aloe vera gel or vaseline gauze. The average healing time for gauze patients was 18 days. The average healing time for aloe vera patients was 12 days.

- Miller, M. B., Koltai, P. J. (1995). Treatment of experimental frostbite with pentoxifylline and aloe vera cream. *Archives of Otolaryngological Head and Neck Surgery*, **121**(6): 678–80.

Experiments were carried out on New Zealand white rabbits and tissue survival was used as a marker for comparison. The untreated group had 6% tissue survival. The pentoxifylline and aloe vera groups had tissue survivals of 20% and 24% respectively. Best results were obtained when both treatments were used together (30% tissue survival).

Mechanism of action

Aloe vera contains over 75 known constituents and more are being discovered regularly. The main groups of chemicals include:

- Vitamins: antioxidant vitamins E, C and beta-carotene, and vitamin B_{12}.
- Minerals and trace elements: selenium, sodium, potassium, calcium, chromium, manganese, magnesium, zinc and copper.
- Amino acids: 20 of the 22 amino acids (7 of the 8 essential amino acids).

- Digestive enzymes.
- Fatty acids: anti-inflammatory.
- Sugars: mucopolysaccharides, e.g. mannose 6-phosphate, may act as active growth substances.
- Saponins: antimicrobial activity.
- Anthraquinones: antimicrobial and analgesic properties.

The properties of these constituents – protection from free radicals, promotion of epithelial wound healing, antimicrobial activity and anti-inflammatory effects – appear to contribute significantly to the overall benefits of aloe vera therapy.

WHICH CONDITIONS ARE SUITABLE FOR TREATMENT WITH ALOE VERA?

- Skin: eczema, dermatitis
                                         psoriasis
                                         ulcers, e.g. infective ulcers,
                                         pressure sores
                                         acne
                                         burns

- Gastrointestinal problems: irritable bowel syndrome
                                         colitis (as an adjunct to
                                         conventional therapy)
                                         diverticulitis

- Post-viral fatigue syndrome

- Arthritis: osteoarthritis
                                         rheumatoid arthritis (as an adjunct
                                         to conventional therapy)

- Prevention: aloe vera is being increasingly recommended by complementary practitioners as a method of helping disease prevention and health promotion

WHICH CONDITIONS ARE NOT SUITABLE FOR TREATMENT WITH ALOE VERA?

- Any condition that may be caused by serious underlying disease

- Serious infections

Advantages

- Natural.
- Safe.
- No side-effects.
- Useful source of vitamin B_{12} for vegetarians and vegans.
- Increasing research is being carried out on its constituents and effects.
- Does not interact with patient's existing medication.

Disadvantages

- Cost.
- Pure aloe vera products may be difficult to obtain.
- Many companies have started to market products with 'aloe vera added'. It is unlikely that the modest amount of aloe vera actually present is of any benefit.

How much?

A litre of aloe vera juice or gel costs approximately £16.50 (1996 UK price).

Self-help

Aloe vera is available as juice, gels and creams. Toiletry and beauty products are also available.

The International Aloe Science Council (IASC) monitors the quality and quantity of aloe in products. Look for its seal of approval.

Vitamin E

Background

Some of the recent claims for vitamin E have been its protective effects against ischaemic heart disease, cancer, rheumatoid arthritis and cataracts. It may even influence the ageing process. Vitamin E is able to exert these effects by its favourable interaction with *free radicals* – molecular fragments containing a free electron.

Free radicals are a normal by-product of aerobic metabolism. They are also produced on exposure to cigarette smoke, X-rays, sunlight and ozone. By gaining or donating electrons in cellular chemical reactions these molecular fragments induce chain reactions which produce more free radicals. In ischaemic heart disease free radicals are thought to cause narrowing of the coronary arteries by encouraging deposition of cholesterol into the artery wall. Malignant change and tumour growth may be caused by free radical attack on cell DNA. Other degenerative diseases could be triggered by free radical interference with biochemical processes.

To protect itself against these harmful effects the body uses antioxidants to scavenge free radicals. Antioxidants are compounds that are able to donate electrons and hydrogen without becoming free radicals themselves. Vitamin E is one of a range of such protective antioxidants. Vitamin C and beta-carotene have a similar effect. Some enzymes containing or depending on the presence of trace elements selenium, zinc, copper and manganese are also thought to be involved in mopping-up free radicals.

Research

- Riemepa, R. A., Wood, D. A., MacIntyre, C. C. *et al.* (1991). Risk of angina pectoris and plasma concentrations of vitamins A, C, E and carotene. *Lancet*, **337**(8732): 1–5.

A prospective study of 6,000 men in Edinburgh. Men with low levels of vitamin E and C and beta-carotene were three times at risk of developing angina compared with those with normal levels.

- Meir, J., Stampfer, M. D., Henneke, C. H. *et al.* (1993). Vitamin E consumption and the risk of coronary disease in women. *The New England Journal of Medicine*, **328**(20): 1444–9.

A prospective study of 87 000 American female nurses. For women taking vitamin E supplements for 2 years, the risk of cardiovascular disease was reduced by a third. The risk was reduced to a half if the supplement was taken for longer.

- Rimm, E. B., Meir, J., Stampfer, M. D. *et al.* (1993). Vitamin E consumption and the risk of coronary heart disease in men. *The New England Journal of Medicine*, **328**(20): 1450–6.

A prospective study of 40 000 American male doctors. The risk of cardiovascular disease was reduced by a quarter after taking vitamin E supplements for more than 2 years.

- Stephens, N. G., Parsons, A., Schofield, P. M. *et al.* (1996). Randomised controlled trial of vitamin E in patients with coronary disease: Cambridge Heart Antioxidant Study (CHAOS). *Lancet*, **347**(9004): 781–6.

In patients with angiographically proven symptomatic coronary atherosclerosis, vitamin E therapy substantially reduces the rate of non-fatal myocardial infarction, with beneficial effects after one year of treatment.

Mechanism of action

Vitamin E is an antioxidant; it works with vitamin C to prevent free radical oxidation of low-density lipoproteins and very low density lipoproteins (LDL/VLDL) – the main carriers of harmful cholesterol in the blood. These oxidized lipids are deposited in arterial walls causing atherosclerosis.

WHICH CONDITIONS ARE SUITABLE FOR TREATMENT WITH VITAMINE E?

- People at risk of cardiovascular disease:
    overweight
    smokers
    high cholesterol levels
    familial hypercholesterolaemia (family history of high cholesterol levels)
    history of ischaemic heart disease (heart attack, angina)

WHICH CONDITIONS ARE NOT SUITABLE FOR TREATMENT WITH VITAMIN E?

- Blood clotting disorders
- Vitamin K deficiency

Advantages

- Safe.
- May prevent degenerative diseases and cancer (but more research needed).

Disadvantages

Much larger studies are needed to determine the optimal dose for preventative therapy. Doses of 40–50 mg are usually recommended.

Simple self-help measures

Patients can obtain adequate amounts of vitamin E by dietary modification and supplements. Patients need about 40–50 mg a day.

- Diet will contribute approximately 20 mg a day, from:
     vegetable oil
     wheat germ (e.g. brown bread)
     leafy vegetables
     egg yolk
     margarine
     legumes (e.g. beans or peas)
- Supplements: some specialists favour a dose of 50 mg daily. Anything else obtained from the diet is a bonus.

How much?

Vitamin E 50 mg costs £5.29 for 100 tablets (1996 UK price).

Garlic

Background

Garlic's medicinal properties have been recognized for centuries. Earliest known records date back to ancient Egypt, where garlic was thought so holy it was invoked as a deity in oaths. In both World Wars it was used to treat gangrene and dysentery. Garlic is extensively used in the Indian subcontinent, China and Southeast Asia, not only for its flavour but also for its health properties. Garlic is often prescribed by complementary practitioners for the prevention and treatment of colds and influenza. Research (see below) now also seems to indicate that garlic may help in maintaining healthy levels of blood fats and cholesterol. For example, taking garlic regularly may:

     inhibit clot formation
     reduce blood pressure
     reduce blood glucose

increase fibrinolysis (the process of removing microscopic blood clots from the circulation)
lower blood fats and cholesterol levels.

The overall effect therefore is to reduce the incidence of athero-sclerosis.

Research

- Sainani, G. S., Desai, D. B., Gorhe, N. H. *et al.* (1979). Effect of dietary garlic and onion on serum lipid profile in a Jain commumity. *Indian Journal of Medical Research*, **69**: 776–80.

Many Jains are prohibited from eating garlic and onions because they are root vegetables. Levels of blood cholesterol were inversely proportional to the levels of consumed garlic.

- Keys, A. (1980). Wine, garlic and CHD (coronary heart disease) in seven countries. *Lancet*, **1**: 145–6.

This European study noted an inverse relationship between garlic consumption and cardiovascular disease.

- Ayer, W., Eiber, A., Hertkorn, E. *et al.* (1990). Hypertension and hyperlipidaemia: garlic helps in mild cases. *British Journal of Clinical Practice*, **44:** (69): 3–7.

In this study, 250 patients with high blood lipid levels were given concentrated garlic powder for 16 weeks. At the end of the therapy period total cholesterol levels were reduced by 12% and triglyceride levels by 17%. There was also a significant reduction in diastolic blood pressure.

- Rassoul, F., Richter, V. and Rotzsch, W. (1992). Total and HDL cholesterol screening in the town of Leipzig: influence of diet and Allium sativum. *European Journal of Clinical Research*, **3A**: 8–9.

Leipzig, Germany. A total of 1430 patients with moderately high cholesterol were given garlic as a dietary supplement. The results showed garlic to be four times as effective as diet alone in lowering cholesterol.

- McMahon, F. G., Jain, A., Vargas, R. *et al.* (1992). Clinical effects of garlic powder preparation on various cardiovascular risk factors. *European Journal of Clinical Research*, **3A**: 8–9.

New Orleans, USA. Patients with severe hypertension had a significant drop in blood pressure after therapy with garlic tablets.

- De, O. S., Santos, A. and Grunwald, J. (1993). Effect of garlic powder tablets on blood lipids and blood pressure – a six month placebo controlled, double blind study. *British Journal of Clinical Research*, **4**: 37–44.

Effect of garlic powder on blood lipids and blood pressure – a 6-month placebo-controlled, double-blind study. LDL cholesterol levels and both systolic and diastolic blood pressure were significantly reduced after 6 months of treatment.

Mechanism of action

Fresh garlic does not smell until it is cut, crushed or heated. Alliinase released by this process breaks down the amino acid alliin, producing allicin. The latter is responsible for the taste, odour and medicinal properties of garlic.

Allicin appears to work as a protective antioxidant, rather like vitamin E. It inhibits the formation of oxygen free radicals which cause LDL/VLDL cholesterol (one of the main carriers of harmful cholesterol in the blood) to oxidize and be deposited in arterial walls leading to atherosclerosis. Other researchers have postulated that the biosynthesis of cholesterol is reduced by garlic and more specifically the enzyme HMG-CoA-reductase is inhibited.

WHICH CONDITIONS ARE SUITABLE FOR TREATMENT WITH GARLIC?

- High cholesterol levels

- Familial hypercholesterolaemia

- History of ischaemic heart disease (heart attack, angina)

- Influenza, coughs, colds (use garlic raw or as a drink)

Advantages

- Natural.
- Safe.
- Credible research work carried out.

Disadvantages

- Allicin is unstable and rapidly loses its activity. Garlic therefore needs to be taken at regular intervals through the day to provide maximum benefit.
- Odour (but see below).
- Some side-effects:
  burning sensation in the mouth
  burning in the stomach
  occasional nausea.
- High doses (equivalent to two whole heads of garlic) can cause loss of appetite, diarrhoea and vomiting.

How much?

- Garlic therapy using 300-mg tablets (equivalent to 900 mg of fresh bulb):
  1–2 tablets daily
  £13.95 for 100 tablets.
- Garlic therapy using 100-mg tablets (equivalent to 300 mg of fresh bulb):
  2 tablets three times daily
  £8.95 for 200 tablets (1996 UK prices).

Simple self-help measures

Garlic tablets (Kwai) are available over the counter. A special coating stops the unpleasant odour.

Increase the amount of garlic in the diet – raw or used in cooking. To cut down the problem of garlic odour consume with parsley, coriander, salad greens, aromatic seeds or aniseed.

Green-lipped mussel

Background

The various forms of arthritis are a major cause of disability worldwide. Simple analgesics for osteoarthritis and non-steroidal anti-inflammatory drugs (NSAIDs) for rheumatoid arthritis have been the mainstay of treatment. However, such medication is not wholly effective and the side-effects of NSAIDs (e.g. gastrointestinal bleeding), particularly in the elderly, remain a problem.

The green-lipped mussel (*Perna canaliculus*), farmed in the unpolluted waters off the New Zealand coast, may provide a viable alternative to conventional treatment. Regular amounts of green-lipped mussel extract taken in capsule form by arthritis sufferers has several beneficial effects, reducing pain and stiffness and improving the sufferer's quality of life.

Research

- Gibson, R. G., Gibson, S. L. M., Conway, V. *et al.* (1980). Perna canaliculus in the treatment of arthritis. *Practitioner*, **224**: 955–60.

This double-blind cross-over study at the Glasgow Homoeopathic Hospital suggested that green-lipped mussel extract was an effective supplement and possibly an alternative to conventional medicine in the treatment of osteoarthritis and rheumatoid arthritis.

- Miller, T. and Wu, H. (1984). *In vivo* evidence for prostaglandin inhibitory activity in New Zealand green-lipped mussel extract. *New Zealand Medical Journal*, **97**(755): 355–7.

The prostaglandin inhibitory effects of green-lipped mussel extract were demonstrated on rats. This inhibition is a central activity of conventional anti-inflammatory products such as aspirin and ibuprofen.

Mechanism of action

As well as their action on innumerable biological processes and metabolism, prostaglandins also play an important role in inflammatory changes. The therapeutic effect of green-lipped mussel extract is probably due to the presence of a biochemical agent that affects the cyclo-oxygenase enzyme system. This in turn causes prostaglandin inhibition and reduces inflammation.

WHICH CONDITIONS ARE SUITABLE FOR TREATMENT WITH GREEN-LIPPED MUSSEL EXTRACT?

- Rheumatoid arthritis
- Other forms of inflammatory joint disease
- Osteoarthritis

WHICH CONDITIONS ARE NOT SUITABLE FOR TREATMENT WITH GREEN-LIPPED MUSSEL EXTRACT?

- High blood pressure (the extract contains natural sea salts)

Advantages

- Natural.
- Safe.
- Viable alternative or supplement to conventional treatment.
- Credible research done.

Disadvantages

- Contraindicated in allergy to shellfish or gelatin.
- Occasional increase in pain in the first few days.
- Slight fishy odour of capsules.

How much?

Green-lipped mussel extract capsules (Seatone):

230-mg capsules, 4 capsules daily – £10.19 for 110 capsules.
350-mg capsules, 3 capsules daily – £4.59 for 30 capsules, £11.19
for 90 capsules (1996 UK prices).

The dose of mussel extract required to maintain improvement varies from patient to patient. Most patients require a minimum of 700 mg daily.

Address for information

Dietary Specialities Ltd
Burford House
179–181 Lower Richmond Road
Richmond
Surrey TW9 4LN

Folic acid

Background

Taking folic acid during the first 12 weeks of pregnancy reduces the risk to the body of neural tube defects – spina bifida ('split spine') and anencephaly (absence of most of the brain). About 800 pregnancies a year are affected in England and Wales. The vast majority result in termination.

Since 1992 the UK Department of Health has recommended that women planning a pregnancy should increase their folic acid intake by 400 micrograms (μg) a day. Women who have had an affected pregnancy can reduce the risk of recurrence by almost 70% by taking 5 mg of folic acid. Taking 5 mg of folic acid a day is also advised for women on antiepileptic treatment. The lower dose of 400 μg is recommended for women with no previous affected pregnancies. In all cases therapy should ideally be commenced 3 months *before* conception and continued until the twelfth week of pregnancy.

Folic acid may also protect against colonic cancer, cervical 'precancer' and cardiovascular disease.

Research

Numerous well-designed studies have shown a definite preventative benefit of folic acid in women with a previous history of neural tube defects.

Some American studies have revealed that Western women do not eat enough fresh fruit and vegetables, the dietary source of folic acid. In one study up to 15% of women aged 20–44 years showed biochemical evidence of folic acid deficiency.

Mechanism of action

Folic acid is thought to exert its effects by lowering levels of homocysteine, a derivative of the amino acid methionine. Elevated levels of homocysteine have been found in women with recurrent miscarriages and neural tube defects.

WHICH CONDITIONS ARE SUITABLE FOR TREATMENT WITH FOLIC ACID?

- No previous pregnancy affected – 400 μg daily
- Patient with a spina bifida child – 5 mg daily
- Previous neural tube defect pregnancy – 5 mg daily
- Patient on antiepileptic treatment – seek specialist advice

Advantages

- Definite prevention of recurrence of neural tube defects.
- Safe if given by itself.
- Treatment backed by doctors and midwives.

Disadvantages

Sometimes given with multivitamins – danger of vitamin overdose. Folic acid should only be given by itself or with iron (if the expectant mother is anaemic).

How much?

Folic acid is available in the UK in tablet form as:

- 5 mg tablets – prescription only
- 400 μg tablets – available from pharmacists at £3.99 for 90 (1996 UK prices).

Simple self-help measures

- Dietary folate:
    at least 50 μg per 56 g serving in –
        asparagus
        brussels sprouts
        black-eyed beans
        beef extract
        yeast extract
        kale
        spring greens
        broccoli
        green beans
        spinach

15 μg to 50 μg per serving –
potatoes
fresh fruit
vegetables
most nuts
tahini
orange juice
baked beans
bread
eggs
milk and milk products
brown rice
wholegrain pasta
salmon, beef, game.
- Avoid irradiated food – irradiation destroys folic acid.
- Fortified foods:
  approximately 50% of breakfast cereals
  approximately 10–20% of breads
  give up to 100 μg per serving (check label).

Fasting

Background

Fasting is an important component of many of the world's religions, for example the Muslim month of Ramadan and the Christian period of Lent. Unlike starvation, fasting can be viewed as a time of rest for the body. Instead of having to expend energy in the breakdown of food and its absorption, the body is able to divert some of these resources to eliminate toxins and restore homoeostasis. When fasting is part of a religious process it is associated with abstinence from not only food but also anger, impiety, profanity and falsehood – 'toxins of the psyche'.

Fasting need not be total. Mono-diets where one food or type of food (usually fruit or vegetables) is eaten for a given period are becoming more popular. The Hindu religion incorporates such mono-diets where a person may live on a particular type of fruit for one day a week.

Research

- Kjeldsen-Kragh, J., Haugen, M., Borchgrevink, C. F. et al. (1991). Controlled trial of fasting and one-year vegetarian diet in rheumatoid arthritis. Lancet, **338**: 899–902.

Twenty-seven patients suffering from rheumatoid arthritis fasted 7–10 days. Patients were then placed on an individual gluten-free vegan diet (i.e. no meat, eggs or dairy products) for 3–5 months. A control group of 26 patients ate a normal diet. The fasting and vegan diet group showed promising results: less pain, fewer tender joints, less morning stiffness and better grip strength.

Mechanism of action

The beneficial effects of fasting are believed to derive from the elimination of toxins and the exclusion of allergens. Fasting is a 'rest' for the bowel.

WHICH CONDITIONS ARE SUITABLE FOR TREATMENT BY FASTING?

- Obesity
- Familial hypercholesterolaemia
- High cholesterol levels

WHICH CONDITIONS ARE NOT SUITABLE FOR TREATMENT BY FASTING?

- Any medical ailment requiring regular medication (e.g. diabetes, ischaemic heart disease)
- Pregnancy
- Children under 12 years of age

Advantages

- Simple to plan.
- Cheap.

Disadvantages

- Nutritional deficiencies occur if fasting is too long and too strict.

5

Postural therapies

Alexander technique

Background

Frederick M. Alexander was born in Tasmania in 1869. His work as a Shakespearean actor of some repute was troubled by hoarseness towards the end of long monologues. Having had no luck with the medical profession he elected to investigate the ailment himself. After years of laborious observation (by three-way mirrors) and experimentation he came to the conclusion that the problem with his vocal cords was related to maladaptive posture and movement of the *whole* body: he was squeezing his vocal cords by pulling his head back and down and shortening his spine. Once these 'habitual poses' were overcome by concentration and exercise, Alexander's voice and general health improved remarkably.

Alexander taught both in the UK and America until 1955. His most famous pupil was Aldous Huxley, who gave Alexander much publicity in the 1920s.

Research

No major study has been carried out on the Alexander technique.

Mechanism of action

Proprioceptors are nerve endings in joints and muscles which provide information on the body's orientation in space. Increased awareness of proprioceptive stimuli allows greater understanding of body function and eventual correction of inappropriate posture and movement.

Patients need to learn to stop wrong habitual movements; these movements become reflex actions, and people do not give themselves time to consider how they will proceed. As Alexander said, 'If we will stop the wrong thing, the right thing does itself'. Patients do not work directly for the end but attend only to the means for achieving it (for example, Alexander concentrated on the correct position of head, neck and spine; his voice improved automatically).

The techniques

A brief history of the medical problem (if present) is taken. The patient (or pupil) remains fully clothed.

Practitioners teach the pupil *how* to change the ingrained faults and habits of a lifetime. Lying on a couch, the pupil is taught 'inhibition': the practitioner (or teacher) moves a part of the body passively. The initial response from the pupil is to reflexly resist this movement. With the help of the teacher the patient works to inhibit this response.

Once this concept of inhibition is understood, pupils are taught how to use their body correctly and inhibit the old habits of incorrect movement and posture. For instance, standing up correctly: the teacher may hold the head and the back between the shoulder blades. The pupil will stand and sit using the correct technique, i.e. using the legs for power and *not* leading with the head.

Breath control and breathing techniques are also taught to aid easier and more efficient movement.

WHICH CONDITIONS ARE SUITABLE FOR TREATMENT BY THE ALEXANDER TECHNIQUE?

- Pain relief: back pain
                      sciatica
                      myalgia (muscle aches)
                      whiplash
                      repetitive strain injury

- Psychological: stress, tension
                      anxiety
                      insomnia

- Pregnancy: back pain

- Allergies: asthma

- Poor posture

- Chronic conditions: multiple sclerosis
                                 Parkinson's disease

- Help in breathing and voice
  control in: singers
                                 dancers
                                 public speakers
                                 actors

- Sports injuries: aid in rehabilitation

WHICH CONDITIONS ARE NOT SUITABLE FOR TREATMENT BY THE ALEXANDER TECHNIQUE?

- Any condition that may be caused by serious underlying disease
- Serious infections

Advantages

- Safe.
- Can enhance general well-being, posture and breathing as well as helping specific ailments.
- Courses often organized by local authorities in day or evening classes. Sports centres, fitness clubs and health farms may also offer courses.
- Patients and pupils are able to learn the technique and to practise it without the presence of a teacher.
- Increasing demand for teachers of the technique.

Disadvantages

- Not available on the NHS.
- Time and cost. A full course will take 2–3 months (see below).
- Some confusion as to whether it is a therapy or a science.

How long and how much?

First session: 1 hour.
Subsequent sessions: 30 minutes to 1 hour.
How many sessions? 20–30 in a complete course, taking 2–3 months to complete. Teachers recommend refresher courses at regular intervals.
Cost: £15–25 (1996 UK prices).

NHS or private? (applicable to the UK only)

- **NHS:** the Alexander technique is not available on the NHS.
- **Private:** teachers and therapists are easily located. Many courses are available locally. Refer only to members of professional organizations.

Address for referral

Society of Teachers of Alexander
Technique (STAT)
20 London House
266 Fulham Road
London SW10 9EL
Tel. 0171 351 0828

Addresses for education and training

Alexander Teaching Centre
188 Old Street
London EC1 9BP
Tel. 0171 250 3038

Alexander Technique Training Centre
Community College
Fore Street
Totnes
Devon TQ9 5RP
Tel. 01803 864218

Centre for the Alexander Technique
46 Stevenage Road
London SW6 6HA
Tel. 0171 731 6348

Constructive Teaching Centre
18 Lansdowne Road
London W11 3LL
Tel. 0171 727 7222

Mcdonald Training Course for the
Alexander Technique
50A Belgrave Road
London SW1
Tel. 0171 821 7916

New Alexander School
21 Lyndhurst Road
Hampstead NW3 5NX
Tel. 0171 435 4321

North London Alexander School
10 Elmcroft Avenue
London NW11
Tel. 0181 455 3938

School of Alexander Studies
44 Park Avenue North
London NW8
Tel. 0181 348 5054

Feldenkrais technique

Background

The Feldenkrais technique is a synthesis of Alexander technique, yoga, stretching and Eastern martial arts. It was developed by Moshe Feldenkrais, an atomic physicist, after he had injured his knee during a judo session. In addition to the pursuit of basic Alexander technique philosophy (i.e. stopping habitual poor posture and movement and encouraging natural motion), Feldenkrais also believed that there was a similar change in habitual (and restrictive) mental attitudes – *body psychotherapy* is a name sometimes given to this technique.

The essential difference between the Alexander and the Feldenkrais techniques is that the former deals with the body in space, whereas the latter is concerned with the body in motion. Pupils follow the teacher's lead of simple, basic natural movement – rather like *t'ai chi*. Teaching on a one-to-one basis is also given (like the Alexander technique) to guide pupils through their methods of movement.

Research

- Ruth, S. and Kegerreis, S. (1992). Facilitatiing cervical flexion using a Feldenkrais method: awareness through movement. *Journal of Orthopaedic and Sports Physical Therapy*, **16**(1): 25–9.

Thirty normal subjects who performed a Feldenkrais exercise attained more neck flexibility than those who sat and chose their own activity (e.g. reading, listening to music, etc.).

This study would have been more useful if it had compared Feldenkrais with another technique, e.g. physiotherapy, ultrasound.

Mechanism of action

Proprioceptors are nerve endings in joints and muscles which provide information on the body's orientation in space. Increased awareness of proprioceptive stimuli allows greater understanding of body function and eventual correction of inappropriate posture and movement.

Each natural movement (walking, crawling, turning the head, bending, etc.) is broken down into its constituent parts. These are incorporated into simple exercises taught in groups.

Freedom from restrictive and habitual postures may allow more mental freedom and change in mental attitudes and outlook.

The techniques

A basic physical history and examination are required if the pupil
has an ailment. The pupil remains fully clothed.

Group work
The pupils follow the teacher through a series of simple movements.

Individual work
Pupils are taught how to use their bodies correctly and inhibit the
'old habits' of incorrect movement and posture. For example, bending and lifting correctly: the teacher may guide the pupil by giving a
series of instructions with the occasional placing of hands:

'*Let* your neck be free'
'*Let* your head go forward and up'
'*Let* your back lengthen and widen'
'*Let* your head move forward'
'*Let* your knees bend'
'*Let* your hips move backwards'.

Breathing
Breath control and breathing techniques are also taught to aid
easier and more efficient movement.

**WHICH CONDITIONS ARE SUITABLE FOR TREATMENT
BY THE FELDENKRAIS TECHNIQUE?**

- Pain relief: back pain
                        sciatica
                        myalgia (muscle aches)
                        whiplash
                        repetitive strain injury

- Psychological: stress, tension
                        anxiety
                        insomnia

- Pregnancy: back pain

- Allergies: asthma

- Poor posture

- Chronic conditions: multiple sclerosis
                        Parkinson's disease

- Help in breathing and voice control in singers, dancers, public speakers and actors
- Sports injuries: aid in rehabilitation
- Used by athletes for: increased functional integration
                          increased understanding of
                          human dynamics
                          better mental attitude

WHICH CONDITIONS ARE NOT SUITABLE FOR TREATMENT BY THE FELDENKRAIS TECHNIQUE?

- Any condition that may be caused by serious underlying disease
- Serious infections

Advantages

- Safe.
- Can enhance general well-being, posture and breathing as well as helping specific ailments.
- Patients and pupils are able to learn technique and practise without a qualified teacher present.

Disadvantages

- Not available on the NHS.
- Time and cost.
- Some confusion as to whether it is a therapy or a science.
- Popular in the USA, but few practitioners in the UK.

How long and how much?

First session: 1 hour.
Subsequent sessions: 30 minutes to 1 hour.
How many sessions? 20–30 in a complete course, taking 2–3 months to complete. Teachers recommend refresher courses at regular intervals.
Cost: £15–25 (1996 UK prices).

NHS or private? (applicable in the UK only)

- **NHS:** Feldenkrais therapy is not available on the NHS.
- **Private:** practitioners are more difficult to locate than those practising the Alexander technique.

Addresses for referral, education and training

The Feldenkrais Guild UK
PO Box 370
London N10 3XA

The Feldenkrais Guild
524 Ellsworth Street
Albany, OR 97321
USA
Tel. 800 775 2118/541 926 0981

6

Psychosomatic therapies

Hypnotherapy

Background

On the whole people are familiar with hypnosis as a form of entertainment, performed by a sinister figure with penetrating eyes, swinging a watch on a chain. The patient, once under 'the influence', is then imbued with superhuman powers or does something unexpected and outrageous on a given cue.

Like other complementary therapies such as acupuncture or homoeopathy, hypnosis has a long history. Anton Mesmer (1734–1815), an Austrian physician, was the founder of hypnosis as we know it. Apart from hypnosis his other not inconsiderable talents included playing the glass harmonica, and the claim that he was Mozart's number one fan. John Elliotson (1791–1868), professor of medicine at University College Hospital, London, not only introduced the stethoscope to England but also hypnosis or 'mesmerism' as it was then called.

James Braid (1795–1860) started experimenting with hypnosis after a public demonstration and suggested the name 'hypnotism' after the Greek word meaning 'sleep'. At about the same time, James Esdaile while working for the East India Company performed over 300 major operations (mainly excision of scrotal tumours) on hypnotized patients.

Sigmund Freud (1856–1939) began to use hypnosis in his psychoanalytical therapy. He demonstrated beyond all doubt that the unconscious mind held prisoner a host of memories that had slipped from the conscious mind, and that although they were forgotten they could have an enormous effect on the behaviour of the individual. He further showed that these repressed memories could be recalled in psychoanalysis and hypnosis and that the effect of this purging or catharsis would frequently result in a cure of the condition.

Hypnosis was used frequently in both World Wars to treat shell-shock. Some say that its use in this field is now undisputed.

The use of hypnosis as a means of analgesia and general therapy declined dramatically after World War II because it failed to gain recognition from the medical profession as a whole. Hypnosis has recently seen an upsurge of interest in the UK largely due to the huge popularity of television stage hypnotists in action amongst a studio audience. Apart from its entertainment value, hypnosis has a great deal to contribute to modern medicine.

Research

- Maher-Loughman, G. P., MacDonald, N., Mason, A. A *et al.* (1962). Controlled trial of hypnosis in the treatment of asthma. *British Medical Journal*, **2**: 371–6.

Progressive relaxation therapy and hypnosis both reduced asthmatic symptoms; 59% of the hypnosis group were much better compared with 43% of the relaxation group. Hypnosis also reduced the use of drugs and frequency of wheezy attacks.

- Fuchs, K., Paldi, E., Abramovici, H. *et al.* (1980). Treatment of hyperemesis gravidarum by hypnosis. *International Journal of Clinical and Experimental Hypnosis*, **28**: 313–23.

In 138 patients with severe vomiting in pregnancy not helped by medication, hypnosis helped 88%.

- Holroyd, J. (1980). Hypnosis treatment for smoking: an evaluative review. *International Journal of Clinical and experimental Hypnosis*, **4**: 341–57.

Seventeen studies were reviewed. The programmes which included hypnosis as well as follow-up had success rates of over 50%.

- Cochrane, G. and Friesen, J. (1986). Hypnotherapy in weight loss treatment. *Journal of Consulting and Clinical Psychology*, **54**: 489–92.

Two groups of obese patients received hypnosis only or hypnosis and an audiotape. A control group of obese patients received 'attention' only. Both hypnosis groups lost an average of 17 pounds in 6 months. The control group put on half a pound.

- Haanen, H. C. M., Hoenderdos, H. T. W., van Romunde, L. K. J. *et al.* (1991). Controlled trial of hypnotherapy in the treatment of refractory fibromyalgia. *Journal of Rheumatology* **18**(1): 72–5.

Patients undergoing hypnosis reported less pain and fatigue compared with those who received physiotherapy.

- Echterling, L. G. and Whalen, J. (1995). Stage hypnosis and public lecture effects on attitudes and beliefs regarding hypnosis. *American Journal of Clinical Hypnosis*, **38**(1): 13–21.

Two hundred and five college students participated. Stage hypnosis and lectures increased attendees' motivation to use hypnosis in treatment and decreased belief that hypnotizable individuals are less intelligent. The lecture increased belief that hypnotizability may be linked with creativity and inner strength. Also lectures reduced belief that a hypnotized person is robot-like and automatically acts on all suggestions whereas stage hypnosis increased this belief.

- Lu, D. P. and Lu, G. P.(1996). Hypnosis and pharmacological sedation for medically compromised patients. *Compendium of Continuing Education in Dentistry*, **17**(11): 32, 34–6, 38–40.

In elderly patients or those with cardiac, kidney, liver or other severe systemic disease, hypnosis effectively allows for a reduction in the sedative dose and provides successful and comfortable dental treatment.

Mechanism of action

Bernard Gindes (1953) actually gave a hypnotic formula and stated that if carried out correctly hypnosis must follow:

$$\text{misdirected attention} + \text{belief}$$
$$+ \text{expectation} + \text{imagination} = \text{hypnosis}$$

Misdirected attention is essential so that the subject's attention is concentrated upon something irrelevant to the actual hypnosis. As we will see, every induction technique does this, by using a coin, a fantasy or a watch, etc. While mentally focused on the 'diverting channel', the patient is unable to harbour doubt. Imagination brings together belief and expectation into an irresistible force.

   Hypnosis is often described as a condition being akin to sleep but not actual sleep. The patient is never unconscious. It may be better described as a condition of considerably *increased suggestibility*. Patients who request the therapy allow themselves to be hypnotized.

Uncomfortable sensations such as pain may be assigned to a separate level of consciouness that is distinct from central awareness. Compare this to driving a car: the patient is not aware of every sensation and action that is taking place, in the same way that a driver is unaware of the actions of driving.

Hypnosis may enhance nervous system inhibitory processes that attenuate pain.

Scientific training and an analytical mind are drawbacks to success. It is fatal during hypnosis to stop and think why you are feeling sleepy or why your arm is rising.

The techniques

A brief history of the ailment is taken. Most hypnotists will emphasize that hypnosis is not a cure – rather, it helps patients to help themselves.

Induction techniques

There are almost as many induction techniques as there are practitioners. However, there are a few techniques practised by most hypnotists. The particular one used depends on the practitioner's experience and the personality type of the patient. An induction technique involving a vivid imagination is unlikely to succeed in a subject with poor visual imagery. It may be wiser to choose the 'dropped coin' technique (see below).

- **Arm levitation:** the practitioner induces the subject's arm to move and the hand to caress the face. The arm then drops down to the lap and the subject sinks further into the relaxed state.
- **Eye fixation:** the patient's gaze is fixed on an object (e.g. a watch, a circle, a point on the ceiling) while the practitioner speaks.
- **Picture visualization:** this method is particularly suitable for children who spend much of their time playing in a world of fantasy. It can be equally well applied to adults. The subject is asked to think of a favourite picture, scene, TV programme or image to help induce the hypnotic state.
- **Visual imagery:** the subject is asked to imagine a blackboard with a box of chalk and a duster. The subject is asked to draw something simple on the board and then rub it out. Many patients actually draw in thin air during this technique – a good sign of a deep trance.

- **The coin technique ('dropped coin'):** the patient holds a coin to concentrate on and feel while being talked through the hypnotic state. When the coin drops the subject's eyes will close and the body will go limp.
- **Relaxation through release of tension:** the practitioner asks the patient to tense different parts of the body while being induced, for example to press a foot firmly on the ground or hold an arm rigid. The patient is then asked to quickly release the tension, which should give a feeling of relaxation, rather as a stretched-out rubber band relaxes when let go.
- **Eye closure:** the subject tries to relax deeply with closed eyes while the practitioner induces a trance by a spoken commentary.
- **Counting:** induction also makes use of certain methods for deepening the hypnotic trance such as counting numbers, deep breathing, and limb tension and relaxation. Thus the hypnotist may say, 'You are comfortable and relaxed in your chair. As you sit with your hands lying easily in your lap, start counting slowly back from five to one. With each number you will feel yourself relaxing more and more. Gradually the numbers will become fainter and fainter so that by the time you reach one you will barely be able to say the number. Your eyes will close and your whole body will sink down deeply into the chair. You will feel completely at rest and absolutely relaxed.' The hypnotist speaks in a slow, monotonous tone while repeating key sentences to reinforce the suggestion.

Stages of hypnosis
During the induction the subject will usually move through definite stages of hypnosis – light trance, medium trance and deep or somnambulistic trance. During the actual hypnotic state there is great relaxation, increased suggestibility and an alteration in muscle activity. While the patient is in the trance a further more detailed history is taken to gain a deeper insight into the patient's problem.

In the post-hypnotic state the patient may 'suffer' from amnesia or any one of the numerous suggestions implanted during the trance such as hallucinations or sensory phenomena (e.g. an itchy nose).

Abuse of the technique of hypnotherapy either by the practitioner or a third party is very rare. The protection of the subject lies in the fact that only if the subconscious mind of an individual in hypnosis accepts a suggestion that is compatible with the moral and ethical codes of the individual will the conscious mind be unable to over-ride it.

Some patients may be regressed down the years to an age where a particular traumatic event took place. Post-hypnotic suggestion and regression are two of the most useful ways of helping patients.

WHICH CONDITIONS ARE SUITABLE FOR TREATMENT BY HYPNOTHERAPY?

- Psychological:

  phobias
  stress, anxiety, panic attacks
  asthma
  insomnia
  depression
  relationship problems
  functional sexual problems
  weight disorders

- Learning and performance:

  shyness
  blushing
  concentration
  studying
  examination nerves
  public speaking
  stage fright
  selling
  sports
  driving test

- Addictions:

  smoking
  alcoholism

- Habits:

  nail-biting
  thumb-sucking
  bed-wetting
  overeating
  stuttering

- Obesity

- Pain:

  reduction and control of painful
  conditions such as arthritis,
  cancer

- Pregnancy:

  increased relaxation
  pain reduction
  nausea
  sickness
  heartburn

WHICH CONDITIONS ARE NOT SUITABLE FOR TREATMENT BY HYPNOTHERAPY?

- Any condition that may be caused by serious underlying disease
- Serious infections
- Serious psychiatric illness, e.g. schizophrenia

Advantages

- Safe.
- Non-invasive.
- Popular with the general public.
- Many patients are able to carry out self-hypnosis.
- Good, reputable training available in most parts of the UK.

Disadvantages

- Use on stage as a form of entertainment may have diminished the credibility of hypnosis as a complementary therapy.
- Many patients worry they may do things in a trance that they would not normally wish to.
- Need to trust the therapist completely – some patients may find this difficult.
- Not suitable for very young children or those with a learning or mental disability.
- Cost may be prohibitive for some.

How long and how much?

First session: up to 1 hour.
Subsequent sessions: 30 minutes to 1 hour.
How many sessions? Occasionally one will do. Usually four to six are recommended.
Cost: £20–40 per session (1996 UK prices).

NHS or private? (applicable in the UK only)

- **NHS:** more doctors and paramedical staff are learning hypnosis. Many general practitioners, obstetricians, midwives, pain specialists and dentists use it to reduce pain.
- **Private:** widely available. Refer preferably to those with clinical psychology training or medical qualifications.

Addresses for referral

American Society of Clinical Hypnosis
2200 East Devon Avenue
Des Plaines, IL 60018
USA
Tel. 847 297 3317

Association of Qualified Curative
Hypnotherapists
10 Balaclava Road
Kings Heath
Birmingham B14 7SG
Tel. 0121 444 5435

British Hypnotherapy Association
67 Upper Berkeley Street
London W1
Tel. 0171 723 4443

British Society of Medical and Dental
Hypnotists
73 Ware Street
Hertford SG13 7ED
Tel. 0181 385 7575

Central Register of Advanced
Hypnotherapists
28 Finsbury Park Road
London N4 2JX
Tel. 0171 359 6991

National Council of Psychotherapists
and Hypnotherapy Register
46 Oxhey Road
Oxhey
Watford WD1 4QQ

National Register of Hypnotherapists
and Psychotherapists
12 Cross Street
Nelson
Lancashire
Tel. 01282 699378

Addresses for education and training

British Society of Medical and Dental
Hypnotists
(Address above; courses for doctors and
dentists only)

National College of Hypnotherapy and
Psychotherapy
12 Cross Street
Nelson
Lancashire
Tel. 01282 699378

National School of Hypnosis and
Advanced Psychotherapy
28 Finsbury Park Road
London N4 2JX
Tel. 0171 359 6991

Autogenic therapy

Background

Sometimes referred to as 'Western yoga', autogenics is a method of learning to control voluntary muscles and the body's homoeostatic processes using a form of deep relaxation exercises. The basic concepts of autogenics were first developed by Dr Johannes Schultz, a physician and practising hypnotist, in the late 1920s. He noticed that patients entering the hypnotic state experienced heaviness in the limbs and a general body warmth. They became relaxed and 'passively aware'. Schultz devised a system of relaxation exercises that, once taught, could enable anyone to enter this state of mind and reap the benefits of hypnosis.

Research

- Sargent, J. D., Green, E. E. and Walters, E. D. (1973). Preliminary report on the use of autogenic feedback training in the treatment of migraine and tension headaches. *Psychosomatic Medicine*, **35**(2): 129–35.

In those practising autogenics there was less frequency and less severity of headaches.

- Labbe, E. E. (1995). Treatment of childhood migraine with autogenic training and skin temperature biofeedback. *Headache*, **35**(1): 10–13.

Thirty children aged 7 to 18 years with migraine headaches were involved with the study. 80% of the skin temperature biofeedback plus autogenic training group and 50% of the autogenic training only group showed clinical improvement compared to none of the waiting-list group.

- Many uncontrolled studies have been carried out on therapies related to autogenics, e.g. hypnosis, biofeedback, relaxation and meditation. The majority of orthodox doctors accept the close and intimate links between physical health and mental well-being.

Mechanism of action

Stress, the enviroment and disease have an adverse effect on the body's own self-regulatory homoeostatic processes. Autogenic training helps realign these natural processes and boost immune system function by its effects on brain wave patterns (more alpha and theta waves found in calm, relaxed, dreamy states), the autonomic nervous system (lowering pulse and blood pressure) and higher centres in the cerebral cortex.

The techniques

A brief history is taken of the client's (or trainee's) medical history if an ailment exists, followed by a health questionnaire.

The teacher then carries out a physical and psychological assessment. How motivated is the client? Why does the client wish to learn autogenics?

Intially clients are seen in groups of up to eight persons. The teacher gives the clients simple exercises – 'reclining', 'armchair' and 'simple sitting' – together with correct breathing and relaxation techniques, to make the clients 'passively aware' of their bodies.

At subsequent sessions, six *standard exercises* are taught with emphasis on casual relaxation and passivity. These allow more control over physiological processes.

- Exercise 1: think 'my right arm is heavy', then extend the heaviness to other parts of the body.
- Exercise 2: think 'my hand is warm', then extend the warmth to the other extremities.
- Exercise 3: slows the heart rate.
- Exercise 4: deepens and regularizes the breathing.
- Exercise 5: warms the stomach.
- Exercise 6: cools the forehead.

Intentional exercises are carried out in private by the client, involving release of emotion, natural reaction, aggression, erratic physical movement, etc. – almost a 'temper tantrum'. Clients are encouraged to make a list of situations that cause anger or anxiety and develop strategies to cope with them.

Every session involves a review of the past week's practice.

The teacher and client do not concentrate on the illness – it is assumed that fitness and health will return as the client's skill in autogenics improves.

Advanced autogenics
Advanced autogenics is usually taught to experienced trainees who have a good basic knowledge of the therapy.

- **Autogenic modification:** the client learns to concentrate more specifically, e.g. 'cool the sinuses'.

- **Autogenic meditation:** used for personal development and certain ailments, e.g. insomnia, anxiety.
- **Autogenic neutralization:** looking at the psyche at the same way as autogenics looks at the body, i.e. with 'casual relaxation'.
- **Creativity mobilization technique:** clients clear their thoughts and commence 'mess painting'. As with the intentional exercises described above, emotions and physical movements are allowed out and displayed. This technique allows the release of blocked memories and emotions and increases self-awareness.

WHICH CONDITIONS ARE SUITABLE FOR AUTOGENIC TREATMENT?

- Psychological:

  phobias
  stress, anxiety, panic attacks
  asthma
  irritable bowel syndrome
  insomnia
  depression
  relationship problems
  functional sexual problems

- Learning and performance:

  blushing
  concentration
  studying
  public speaking
  stage-fright
  selling
  sports

- Addictions:

  smoking
  alcoholism

- Habits:

  nail-biting
  thumb-sucking
  bed-wetting
  overeating
  stuttering

- Obesity

- Pain:

  any painful condition –
  reduction and control

- Infertility

- Pregnancy and labour: preparation for childbirth
  increased relaxation
  pain reduction
  nausea
  sickness
  heartburn

- Post-viral fatigue syndrome

- HIV infection, AIDS

- High blood pressure

- Indigestion, peptic ulcers

WHICH CONDITIONS ARE NOT SUITABLE FOR AUTOGENIC TREATMENT?

- Any condition that may be caused by serious underlying disease
- Serious infections
- Serious psychiatric illness, e.g. schizophrenia
- Brittle disease, e.g. asthma or diabetes
- Epilepsy

Advantages

- Safe.
- Non-invasive.
- A strong preventative role. For some, a part of daily living.
- Once taught, clients can use the technique themselves.

Disadvantages

- Time and cost may be prohibitive for some.
- Client may attempt to self-treat an illness that requires orthodox therapy.

How long and how much?

First session: 2 hours.
Subsequent sessions: 2 hours.

How many sessions? seven to ten sessions with a 30-minute daily practice at home. Advanced autogenics will require many more.
Cost: Variable. More expensive in London. Average cost for seven to ten weekly sessions is £160 for group lessons, £300 for individual tuition (1996 UK prices).

NHS or private?

- **NHS:** autogenic training is available at the Royal London Homoeopathic Hospital. Referral can be made by general practitioners who have a contract with the hospital.
- **Private:** easily available. Refer to organizations listed below.

Addresses for referral

British Association for Autogenic
Training and Therapy
18 Holtsmere Close
Watford
Herts WD2 6NG
Tel. 01923 675501

National Childbirth Trust
Alexandra House
Oldham Terrace
London W3
Tel. 0181 992 8637
(For women who wish to use autogenics
for their pregnancy and labour)

Royal London Homoeopathic Hospital
NHS Trust
Great Ormond Street
London WC1N 3HR
Tel. 0171 837 8833

Addresses for education and training

Centre for Autogenic Training
101 Harley Street
London W1Y DF
Tel. 0171 935 1811

Director of Education
Royal London Homoeopathic Hospital
(Address above; training open to GPs,
medical students, nurses, midwives,
pharmacists, veterinary surgeons,
physiotherapists)

Meditation

Background

Meditation is a systematic method of relaxation. The essential difference from relaxation is that it tries to achieve awareness of the body while stilling the conscious and suppressing active thought.

Meditation is associated with many religions. Muslims practise a form of meditation whenever they face Mecca five times a day and recite prayers from the Holy Quran. Followers of Buddhism incorporate forms of meditation into their daily lives. Hinduism particularly has contributed many forms of yoga and meditation (see below). However, meditation can be practised without religious or spiritual associations. In fact most people go through a form of meditation regularly – getting lost in one's own thoughts, being hypnotized by the beauty of a sunset, listening to a piece of music, becoming engrossed in a book, etc.

Systematic meditation takes many forms and there are a number of different philosophies and schools of thought. However, they all have the same goal – to approach and understand higher levels of awareness and to use the experience to gain physical and psychological benefits. For many meditation is not simply a therapy, it is a way of life.

Research

- Lawlis, G. F., Selby, D., Hinnant, D. *et al.* (1985). Reduction of postoperative pain parameters by presurgical relaxation intructions for spinal pain patients. *Spine*, **10**(7): 649–51.

The relaxation group used less analgesia, complained less to nurses and had shorter hospital stays.

- Stuckey, S. J., Jacobs, A. and Goldfarb, J. (1986). Electromyographic (EMG) biofeedback training, relaxation training, and placebo for the relief of chronic back pain. *Perceptual and Motor Skills*, **63**: 1023–36.

Relaxation training was the best method for reducing pain.

- Bridge, L. R., Benson, P., Pietroni, P. C. *et al.* (1988). Relaxation and imagery in the treatment of breast cancer. *British Medical Journal*, **297**(5): 1169–72.

In 154 patients receiving radiotherapy, mood was significantly better in those patients taught relaxation, deep breathing and imagery.

- Whitman, S., Dell, J., Legion, V. *et al.* (1990). Progressive relaxation for seizure reduction. *Journal of Epilepsy*, **3**: 17–22.

Seizure frequency was reduced by over 50% after 6 months of progressive relaxation training.

- Telles, S., Nagarathna, R. and Nagendra, H. R. (1995). Autonomic changes during 'OM' meditation. *Indian Journal of Physiology and Pharmacology*, **39**(4): 418–20.

A statistically significant reduction in heart rate was found amongst meditators during periods of meditation as compared with periods of 'non-targeted' thinking.

- Alexander, C. N., Schneider, R. H., Staggers, F. *et al.* (1996). Trial of stress reduction for hypertension in older African Americans. *Hypertension*, **28**(2): 228–37.

A randomized controlled trial where mental and physical stress reduction approaches (transcendental meditation and progressive muscle relaxation) were compared with a lifestyle-modification, education-control program and with each other. Reductions in blood pressure of the TM group were significantly greater than in the progressive muscle relaxation and lifestyle groups.

- Many uncontrolled studies have been carried out on therapies related to meditation, e.g. hypnosis, biofeedback and relaxation. The majority of orthodox doctors accept the close and intimate links between physical health and mental well-being.

Mechanism of action

Stress, the environment and disease have an adverse effect on the body's own self-regulatory homoeostatic processes. Meditation helps realign these natural processes by its effects on brain wave patterns (more alpha and theta waves found in calm, relaxed, dreamy states), the autonomic nervous system (lowering pulse and blood pressure) and higher centres in the cerebral cortex.

The techniques

The teacher will guide a group of pupils through simple methods of meditation first, moving on later to different techniques to achieve higher planes of awareness or to help with specific ailments.

The basic lessons involve sitting comfortably, learning to relax different muscle groups and breathing exercises. Chants or *mantras* are occasionally used to aid meditation. The most commonly used is *om*. The mantra occupies the mind and the the vibration of sound helps concentrate energy.

Many forms of meditation use sensory stimulation to help develop a particular state, for example by using a picture of a guru or spiritual teacher, a candle flame or flower bud (by concentrating on the image, to try and change its perceived colour, see it grow, open up, etc. – this helps visual perceptive skills). Some stimulate their sense of smell by using aromatic oils or burning incense, others listen to soothing music or the voice of their guru or teacher.

Visualization
The use of imagery has developed into a powerful tool and has clinical applications. 'Directed day-dreaming' or 'guided fantasies' have been used to treat asthma, cancer, ischaemic heart disease and chronic pain. An example is visualization for pain relief – after initial meditation the patient is asked to imagine a dial that can be turned up or down, increasing or decreasing the pain at will.

Transcendental meditation
Popularized by Maharishi Mahesh Yogi in America in the 1970s, transcendental meditation (TM) is based on Hindu teachings, and is achieved through the repetition of a mantra such as *om*.

Pranayama
Pranayama is a form of yoga based on ancient Hindu philosophy. Breathing exercises and control are used to re-balance '*prana*' ('the energy permeating all the universe' – similar to *chi* in Chinese philosophy). Pranayama maintains health and promotes longevity.

Laughing meditation
Laughing meditation can be carried out alone or in groups; it consists of a structured exercise of 15 minutes with three stages – stretching, laughing and silence. Participants often describe feelings of deep relaxation and unburdening.

Meditation requires practice and often regular sessions with a teacher to learn new techniques.

Meditation and related techniques have become so popular that numerous books, tapes, CDs and videos are now available to allow anyone home tuition. Some self-help techniques are described below.

WHICH CONDITIONS ARE SUITABLE FOR TREATMENT BY MEDITATION?

- Psychological:

  phobias
  stress, anxiety, panic attacks
  asthma
  irritable bowel syndrome
  insomnia
  depression
  relationship problems
  functional sexual problems

- Learning and performance:

  blushing
  concentration
  studying
  public speaking
  stage-fright
  selling
  sports

- Addictions:

  smoking
  alcoholism

- Habits:

  nail-biting
  thumb-sucking
  bed-wetting
  overeating
  stuttering

- Obesity

- Pain: any painful condition – reduction and control

- Pregnancy and labour:

  preparation for childbirth
  increased relaxation
  pain reduction
  nausea
  sickness
  heartburn

- Post-viral fatigue syndrome

- HIV infection, AIDS

- High blood pressure

- Indigestion, peptic ulcers

WHICH CONDITIONS ARE NOT SUITABLE FOR TREATMENT BY MEDITATION?

- Any condition that may be caused by serious underlying disease
- Serious infections
- Serious psychiatric illness, e.g. schizophrenia

Advantages

- Safe.
- Non-invasive.
- Popular with the general public.
- A strong preventative role. For some, a part of daily living.
- Many pupils can learn from the numerous books, tapes, CDs and videos available.
- Once taught, clients can use the technique themselves.

Disadvantages

- Time and cost may be prohibitive for some.
- Rarely can cause disorientation, worsened interpersonal relationships, dreamland illusions, unreality, pseudohallucination, increased alienation from society and negativity (therefore not recommended to those predisposed to mental illness).

How long and how much?

First session: up to 1 hour.
Subsequent sessions: 30 minutes to 1 hour.
How many sessions? To learn how to meditate: seven to ten sessions with daily practice at home. Advanced meditation will require many more. For continued benefit aim at two 20-minute sessions daily.
Cost: Varies widely. Minimal cost if self-taught with books and video. A privately-run TM course can cost £400 (1996 UK price).

NHS or private? (applies to the UK only)

- **NHS:** not available on the NHS.
- **Private:** often taught at Buddhist centres, adult education centres or fitness clubs.

Simple self-help techniques

Find a quiet place (you will need 10–20 minutes) and an appropriate chair – comfortable and upright. Sit comfortably, keeping your head, neck and body erect. Close your eyes, and place your hands on your knees. Gradually deepen your breathing: breathe from your stomach; concentrate on gentle inhalation followed by exhalation.

Move your concentration to your forehead: relax your forehead muscles, then gradually work your way down to your eyes, jaw, tongue, shoulders, arms, hands, fingers, chest, abdomen, upper legs, knees, calves, feet and toes. Relax each in turn. Do this slowly and keep breathing smoothly and slowly.

Do not try to banish thoughts that may come; regard them with simple indifference. Concentrate on your breathing.

Music will help deepen the meditation; a chant such as '*om*' or '*who*' (on exhalation) will also help deepen it.

Visualization for relaxation
Once you are comfortable in your chair, close your eyes. Allow a favourite image to develop in your mind – the ocean, a waterfall, mountainside, a painting, etc. Gradually fill in the detail of the picture with colours and objects. Imagine as much detail as you can of each object. Try to include as much sensory stimulation as you can (sights, sounds, smells, touch). Some people ask themselves questions, for example 'Is that the sun I can feel on my back?' 'Can I hear the waterfall?', and so on.

After 10–15 minutes let the image go and bring your attention back to your breathing, your body and eventually to your room.

Addresses for referral

London Zen Society
10 Belmont Street
London NW1
Tel. 0171 485 9576

London Soto Zen Group
23 Westbere Road
London NW2
Tel. 0171 794 3109

Transcendental Meditation
National Communications Office
Tel. 0800 269 303
(For nearest TM centre)

Addresses for education and training

School of Meditation
158 Holland Park Avenue
London W11 4HU
Tel. 0171 603 6116

Transcendental Meditation
National Communications Office
(See above)

Biofeedback

Background

Biofeedback was originally used by psychotherapists as a diagnostic aid, most notably by Carl Jung in the early 1900s. It is a technique that uses sensory information to help control autonomic or involuntary body responses such as blood pressure, skin temperature, pulse, blood flow and peristalsis. Once these physical processes can be controlled they may be used as an aid to relieving certain ailments and maintaining health.

Biofeedback and relaxation are often used together, but there is an important difference between the two. In the former the person focuses on a specific response, e.g. reducing blood pressure. In the latter the aim is to relax the whole body.

The term 'complementary medicine' is well suited to biofeedback since the technique is being increasingly used by the medical profession in research and treatment. However, it may be some time before it is widely available through the NHS.

Research

Biofeedback has a reputable scientific pedigree. Over 2000 papers have been written of which the following are examples.

● Patel, C., Marmet M. G. and Terry D. J. (1981). Controlled trial of biofeedback-aided behavioural methods in reducing mild hypertension. *British Medical Journal*, **282**: 2005–8.

Blood pressure was reduced in patients taught biofeedback and other behavioural methods.

● Rice, B. I. and Schindler, J. V. (1992). Effect of thermal biofeedback-assisted relaxation training on blood circulation in the lower extremeties of a population with diabetes. *Diabetes Care*, **15**(7): 853–8.

Increase in skin temperature will help increase circulation. When diabetics were given a general relaxation tape they were able to increase their toe temperature by 9%. With biofeedback-assisted relaxation the figure was 31%.

● Schleenbacker, R. E. and Mainous III, A. G. (1993). Electromyographic biofeedback for neuromuscular re-education in the hemiplegic stroke patient. *Archives of Physical Medicine and Rehabilitation*, **74**(12): 1301–4.

Biofeedback helped improve hand functions such as grip and grasp. Patients' gait was also improved.

- Iwata, G. *et al.* (1995). New feedback therapy in children with encopresis (faecal soiling due to deliberate intent or psychiatric disorder). *European Journal of Paediatric Surgery*, **5**(4): 231–4.

Biofeedback therapy improved voluntary sphincter function and rectal sensation.

Mechanism of action

The person acquires the skill to consciously alter body processes and systems which are normally under the control of the autonomic nervous system.

The techniques

Electrodes are connected to the skin which can provide information on body systems:

electroencephalograph (EEG)	– brain waves
electromyograph (EMG)	– muscular activity and
	– tension
electrical skin resistance (ESR) meter	– temperature.

This information is translated into audible or visual signals such as bleeps, clicks or waves on a screen. The trainee is then encouraged to use thoughts, sensations, feelings, breath control, meditation and any other means (in a state of relaxation) to alter the signals. People may work on trying to alter the tone or pitch of a sound, the number of clicks per minute, the width of a wave, etc. By giving people this immediate feedback on the state of their internal environment it is possible to teach them how to control it.

Once the state of mind required to change a particular process has been learned the person can detach the electrodes and use the technique anywhere. This is usually more difficult than it seems. Without the benefit of electrode feedback the skill is often quickly lost. To address this problem biofeedback training is being extended, machines are intermittently switched off and often only used to check progress.

WHICH CONDITIONS ARE SUITABLE FOR TREATMENT BY BIOFEEDBACK?

- Pain relief: migraine and chronic headaches
  backache
  neck pain, torticollis
  neuralgia
  chronic or terminal illnesses e.g.
  multiple sclerosis, malignancy
  postoperative pain

- Neurological: Bell's palsy
  Ménière's disease
  vertigo
  stroke

- Psychological: anxiety
  stress
  insomnia
  feeling 'run down'
  post-traumatic stress disorder

- Gynaecological: premenstrual tension
  period pain
  menopausal problems

- Urinary: irritable or unstable bladder
  urinary incontinence

- Allergies: asthma

- Abdominal: irritable bowel syndrome
  faecal incontinence

- Addictions: alcohol, smoking

- Blood pressure

- Raynaud's disease

- Tinnitus

- Diabetes (to improve circulation)

- Post-viral fatigue syndrome

WHICH CONDITIONS ARE NOT SUITABLE FOR TREATMENT BY FIOBEEDBACK?

- Any condition that may be caused by serious underlying disease

- Serious infections

Advantages

- Much credible research done.
- Some of the machinery involved is simple enough to use at home.
- Once taught, can be done anywhere without machines.
- Increasingly recognized by conventional medical practice.

Disadvantages

- Cost of link-up to electrodes and machinery to learn biofeedback may be expensive.
- Dependence on instrumentation. Many find it difficult to practise the therapy without immediate electrode feedback.
- Training and treatment not so readily available as for other complementary techniques.

How long and how much?

First session: $1-1\frac{1}{2}$ hours.
Subsequent sessions: 45 minutes to 1 hour.
How many sessions? Great variation; some patients may need four, others may need over ten sessions. Most patients need regular follow-up to monitor their biofeedback ability.
Cost: £30–40 for $1\frac{1}{2}$ hours. Some patients purchase biofeedback monitors for themselves for regular sessions at home. An ESR meter costs £148 (1996 UK prices).

NHS or private? (applies to UK only)

- **NHS:** not available routinely, although there are some centres that use biofeedback for the treatment of faecal incontinence, strokes, enuresis (bed-wetting) and encopresis.
- **Private:** there are a few reputable centres in the UK that teach or treat with biofeedback.

Addresses for referral

Association for Applied
Psychophysiology and Biofeedback
10200 West 44th Avenue
Wheat Ridge, CO 80033
USA
Tel. 303 422 8436

Biomonitors
2 Old Garden Court
Mount Pleasant
St Albans
Herts AL3 4RQ
Tel. 01727 833882

British Complementary Medicine
Association
9 Soar Lane
Leicester LE3 5DE
Tel. 01162 425406

Institute for Complementary Medicine
PO Box 194
London SE16 1QZ
Tel. 0171 237 5165

Addresses for education
and training

Biomonitors
(Address above)

Institute for Complementary Medicine
(Address above)

7

Sensory therapies

Aromatherapy

Background

Aromatherapy, along with herbal medicine, is perhaps one of the oldest therapies, dating back 6000 years to ancient Egypt and India. It is still used there today. In the last 20 years the therapy has become increasingly popular in Europe, particularly in France, where over 1500 trained doctors occasionally use essential oils as an alternative to antibiotics. It has taken much longer for aromatherapy to be accepted in the UK because it was first introduced in the 1950s as a massage therapy.

Aromatherapy is a natural treatment which uses the aromatic essence of plants to improve and maintain well-being. As with other complementary techniques, therapists have a holistic approach and treat the person as a whole. The oils are extracted from the flowers, leaves, stems and roots of the plant by pressing or solvent extraction. There are some 300 different oils used in aromatherapy. Some can be very expensive due to the rarity of the plant or the fact that a huge amount of plant material yields a very small quantity of oil.

Research

- Shrivastav, P., George, K., Balasubramaniam, N. *et al.* (1988). Suppression of puerpal lactation using jasmine flowers. *Australia and New Zealand Journal of Obstetrics and Gynaecology*, **26**: 68–71.

Women taping jasmine flowers to their breasts in Southern India were able to suppress lactation as well as if they had used bromocriptine.

- Wilkinson, S. (1995). Aromatherapy and massage in palliative care. *International Journal of Palliative Nursing*, **1**(1): 21–30.

Fifty-one cancer patients were given massage either with plain almond oil or an aromatherapy oil. The aromatherapy group reported fewer physical symptoms and less anxiety.

Mechanism of action

The action of aromatherapy on the state of mind depends on the link between smell and memory. Both centres are found in close proximity in the brain which may be why smells and aromas evoke such strong memories. The essential oil aroma stimulates the body into healing itself, working as a catalyst.

Massage and penetration of the oils into the body may also have a direct effect. Different oils have different properties – they may be calming, toning, regulating or stimulating.

The techniques

A full medical history is taken, including personality and possible contraindications to certain oils.

Once a diagnosis has been made the aromatherapist will blend certain oils with a carrier oil (usually wheatgerm, grapeseed or almond oil). The patient is treated as a whole. Different patients may receive different blends for the same condition. The skill of the aromatherapist lies in the blending of the oils and knowing their properties, uses and contraindications.

For home use different techniques may be used:

- Add few drops of oil to bath-water.
- Burn oil in an oil burner.
- Self-massage.
- Use oil as a room scent or perfume.
- Add a few drops to a handkerchief and inhale.
- Add a few drops to a bowl of hot water and inhale the steam.

Occasionally the patient will be prescribed a few drops of oil to ingest daily. Some therapists will also recommend dietary advice and simple exercises.

WHICH CONDITIONS ARE SUITABLE FOR TREATMENT BY AROMATHERAPY?

- Pain relief:
  migraine and chronic headaches
  arthritis (rheumatoid, osteoarthritis)
  cramp
  back pain, sciatica
  neck pain
  muscle strains

- Psychological:
  anxiety
  stress
  insomnia
  feeling 'run down', lethargic
  depression
  anorexia, bulimia

- Allergies:
  asthma
  sinus and catarrhal problems
  urticaria

- Skin:
  eczema
  acne
  cellulite
  psoriasis
  ulcers
  excessive sweating

- Gastrointestinal:
  indigestion
  peptic ulcers
  irritable bowel syndrome
  constipation
  gallstones

- Cardiovascular:
  blood pressure
  varicose veins

- Urinary:
  bed-wetting
  cystitis
  irritable bladder
  kidney stones
  water retention

- Gynaecological:
  premenstrual tension
  menopausal symptoms
  menstrual problems

- Children: behavioural problems
                           colic
                           colds
                           indigestion
                           sleep problems
                           nappy rash
                           teething

- Sports injuries

- Post-viral fatigue syndrome

- Chemotherapy side-effects

- Cancer patients: aid to relaxation, anxiety and pain relief

- Pregnancy: but **avoid certain oils**: i.e. sage, pennyroyal, camphor, parsley, tarragon, wintergreen, juniper, hyssop and basil

WHICH CONDITIONS ARE NOT SUITABLE FOR TREATMENT BY AROMATHERAPY?

- Any condition that may be caused by serious underlying disease

- Serious infections, particularly of the skin

- Severe eczema or psoriasis

- Oil allergies

- Certain oils should be avoided in pregnancy (see above)

Advantages

- Safe.
- Usually non-invasive.
- Increasing in popularity with the general public.
- A portable skill.
- Basic aromatherapy is easily self-taught.
- Plenty of good courses are available locally.

Disadvantages

- Essential oils can be expensive.
- Occasional side-effects such as skin sensitivity.

How long and how much?

First session: 1–2 hours.
Subsequent sessions: 45 minutes.
How many sessions? Occasionally only one is required. Many patients have regular sessions for the massage and relaxation.
Cost: £25–35 per session (1996 UK prices).

NHS or private? (applies to the UK only)

- **NHS:** aromatherapy is increasingly used in cancer patients to help relieve pain, anxiety and stress. Nurses in general are being encouraged to consider the possibility of incorporating aromatherapy and massage along with other complementary techniques into their practice. Some midwives use aromatherapy to help women in labour.
- **Private:** widely available from alternative medicine clinics, fitness clubs and gymnasiums. Refer only to members of professional organizations.

Simple self-help measures

Oils should be kept in dark-coloured containers protected from heat and sunlight. The cost of the pure oil is £3 to £7 depending on the type (1996 UK prices).

Never use aromatic oils 'neat', always mix with a base oil, e.g. almond, sunflower, wheatgerm or avocado. Up to four aromatic oils can be used at once – mix with the base oil in equal quantities. Some essential oils suitable for common ailments are listed in Box 7.1.

- Baths: add 10 drops of oil to the bath-water and soak.
- Inhalation: add 10 drops of oil to a bowl of hot water and inhale.
- Compresses: add 10 drops of oil to 100 ml of hot water. Apply this with a sterile gauze to the affected area.

BOX 7.1 Essential oils for common ailments:

Geranium

premenstrual tension
menopausal symptoms
eczema
acne

Chamomile

stress
eczema

Eucalyptus

sciatica
rheumatism
sore throat
sinusitis

Lavender

migraine, headaches
coughs and colds
during labour
post-natally to reduce perineal discomfort
(bath)
insomnia
anxiety, tension

Ylang-ylang

anger, frustration, irritability
fear

Cypress

varicose veins

Peppermint

cystitis
menopausal symptoms
period pain
indigestion
nausea
headaches

Oils suitable in pregnancy

lavender
orange blossom
rose
geranium

Addresses for referral

Aromatherapy Organisations Council
3 Latymer Close
Braybrooke
Market Harborough
Leics LE16 8LN
Tel. 01858 434242

Association of Tisserand
Aromatherapists
65 Church Street
Hove
East Sussex BN3 2BD
Tel. 01273 772479/206640

British Complementary Medicine
Association
9 Soar Lane
Leicester LE3 5DE
Tel. 01162 425406

International Federation of
Aromatherapists
2–4 Chiswick High Road
London W4 1TH
Tel. 0181 742 2605

Institute for Complementary
Medicine
PO Box 194
London SE16 1QZ
Tel. 0171 237 5165

Register of Qualified Aromatherapists
52 Barracks Lane
Aldwick
Bognor Regis
West Sussex PO21 4DD

**Addresses for education
and training**

Aromatherapy Organisations Council
(Address above)

The Institute for Complementary
Medicine
(Address above)

Association of Tisserand
Aromatherapists
(Address above)

International Federation of
Aromatherapists
(Address above)

Sound therapy

Background

People have used sounds, particularly music, naturally and thera-
peutically through the ages. Egyptian writings over 2500 years old
refer to music and incantations as cures for infertility and rheumatic
pain. Sound therapy was used by the Greeks and the Vedic-Sanskrit
scholars of India. Ayurvedic practitioners in Indian villages still use
it today.

In recent years there has been renewed interest in sound therapy
specifically aimed at organs and general voice therapy in the form of
chants and singing. Some researchers believe that high-frequency
harmonics that many religious chants share may directly affect
various neurophysiological processes.

Research

Although research is being carried out into this therapy no major
studies have yet been published.

Mechanism of action

Each tissue resonates at a particular frequency. Environmental effects, illness and disease cause it to change. The tissue is 're-tuned' by applying a vibration of the same frequency to the body. As the tissue's frequency is corrected, cure is effected.

Sound or voice therapy causes bone vibration which in turn causes the cranium (skull) and the stapes bone of the middle ear to vibrate. Researchers believe the latter may directly stimulate the brain. Psychologically, singing has a significant mood-enhancing effect.

The techniques

After taking a detailed history of the ailment, the therapist will analyse the patient's voice to make a diagnosis, for example:

angry sounding – liver or gallbladder problems
sad sounding – nasal, throat or lung problems
fearful – bladder and urinary problems

Once an ailment has been identified the patient is given a set of chants and mantras to sing in the relevant notes:

- Note C helps poor circulation, anaemia, cold feet.
- Note E helps flatulence, coughs, headaches.
- Note A helps nervousness, shingles, breathing difficulty.

Some therapists may direct sound to parts of the body by making vocalizations themselves near the target organ. Patients are also advised to expose themselves to music and sounds based on these notes.

Patients may be given physical exercises with certain vocalizations to free up and loosen the body (toning); for example:

- Punch the air and stamp on the floor. Then throw your arms up, punch the air again as you utter 'ooh!'.
- Swing your hips slowly saying 'ugh!' with each rotation.

Therapy is often given in groups so that resonance and harmony can help the healing process.

Crystals may be used to augment sound therapy as they are believed to be harmonic resonators. The patient holds the crystal while chanting or singing.

Some sound therapists use ultrasound to deliver the correct frequencies to the affected tissues. This is similar to the treatment given by physiotherapists in sports injuries.

WHICH CONDITIONS ARE SUITABLE FOR TREATMENT BY SOUND THERAPY?

- Any uncomplicated rheumatic condition
- Anxiety, stress, depression
- Headaches
- Fatigue, lack of energy

WHICH CONDITIONS ARE NOT SUITABLE FOR TREATMENT BY SOUND THERAPY?

- Any condition that may be caused by a serious underlying disease
- Serious infections
- Serious psychiatric illness, e.g. schizophrenia

Advantages

- Safe.
- Non-invasive.

Disadvantages

- Cost of treatment is borne by the patient.
- Few practitioners in the UK (but numbers are increasing steadily).

How long and how much?

First session: 1 hour.
Subsequent sessions: 30 minutes to 1 hour.
How many sessions? Variable number, occasionally only one is required.
Cost: £20–30 per session (1996 UK prices).

NHS or private? (applies to the UK only)

- **NHS:** music therapy is often used by physiotherapists as an adjunct to orthodox treatments. It is also used by psychotherapists, particularly those working with children suffering from autism, Down's syndrome and behavioural problems. Day centres for the elderly and infirm play music as an aid to socialization, movement and games.

- **Private:** few practitioners are readily available in the UK. However, the number is steadily increasing.

Simple self-help measures

- Humming, singing regularly: relieves stress, aids relaxation.
- Exaggerated yawning: for tiredness (releases tension in the jaw and mouth).
- Loud groaning or sighing: for irritability, tension.
- Listening to different music and sounds, e.g. sacred chants, Tibetan temple music.

Addresses for referral

Association of Professional Music
Therapists
38 Pierce Lane
Fulbourne
Cambridge CB1 5BL
Tel. 01223 880377

Institute for Complementary Medicine
PO Box 194
London SE16 1QZ
Tel. 0171 237 5165

Ms Susan Lever
2 Woodlea
Coulby Newham
Middlesbrough TS8 0TX
Tel. 01642 590562
(Voice/sound therapy)

Mu Sum Ba Living Rhythm
4 Bramstone Road
London NW10 5TU
(Rhythm and voice work)

Voice Movement Therapist Association
PO Box 4218
London SE22 0JE

Voice Work
6 Goldney Road
Clifton
Bristol BS8 4RB

Addresses for education and training

British Society for Music Therapy
69 Avondale Avenue
East Barnett
Herts EN4 8NB
Tel. 0181 368 8879

Ray Didcock
58 King Georges Avenue
Watford
Herts WD1 7QD
(Workshops on healing sound)

Institute for Complementary Medicine
(Address above)

Nordoff-Robbins Music Therapy
3 Leighton Place
London NW5 2QL
Tel. 0171 267 6296

Ms Susan Lever
The Healing Power of Sound
(Regular workshops, address above)

Prometheus School of Healing
152 Penistone Road
Shelley
Huddersfield
HD8 8JQ
(Sound healing and vibrational
medicine)

Colour therapy

Background

Visible light is made up of the seven colours of the rainbow.
The eyes are sensitive to all the hues in this range but the rest of
the electromagnetic spectrum is invisible. The human body is, however, still sensitive to those energies the eye cannot see, especially
infrared and ultraviolet.

The appreciation of colours and colour therapy was known to
many ancient civilizations, including the Greeks, Romans, Egyptians and Indians. Today it is recognized that colours have a
strong effect on moods and emotions. Colours at the red end of
the spectrum make the body tense and excitable, whereas the blue
end colours are calming and relaxing. Colour also affects our perception. A blue room appears larger than a red one.

Even our language is full of colour analogies such as 'having the
blues', 'green with envy', 'purple with rage', 'seeing red' and the
phrase without which westerns could never have been made –
'yellow-bellied'!

Research

Several uncontrolled studies have shown that exposure to certain
colours can have physiological effects: red light increases pulse,
blood pressure, muscular activity and respiration; blue has the
opposite effect.

Seasonal affective disorder (SAD) – depression brought on by a
lack of sunlight during winter – is often helped by sitting in front
of a full-spectrum light box for a few hours a day. However, this
is more light therapy than colour therapy.

Mechanism of action

Each colour has a characteristic energy level. Disease or illness will cause a deficiency in this energy and hence the colour. Exposure to the corresponding colours will redress this imbalance and reverse the physical and psychological states.

The techniques

The therapist will try to build up a picture of the patient's personality and needs. A personality questionnaire may be filled in. Specifically, the therapist will ask about:

favourite colours
most disliked colours
history of the ailment – to see which colour energies are still strong.

Therapists use several techniques to diagnose which colour energies are lacking; these are described below.

Aura analysis
The human aura is a three-dimensional ovoid. It contains a range of colours which extend from red through orange, yellow, green, turquoise, blue and violet to magenta. Change in shape and colour of a patient's aura (for example flecks or shadows) can indicate minor toxins such as alcohol or nicotine.

Spinal analysis
The spine is divided into five sections, each containing up to eight vertebrae with their different colour energies. The vibrations of the spinal colours can be picked up by 'dowsing' with either a pendulum or a finger. A 'witness' (e.g. a lock of hair, a photograph or a signature from the patient) is placed behind a chart of the spine. The middle finger of the non-dominant hand is slowly moved over the chart. Over the active vertebrae the practitioner will feel a hot, cold or tingling sensation that indicates energy imbalance.

Chakra analysis
Chakras (Figure 7.1) are foci in the body through which energies flow. The eight greater and lesser *chakras* are lens-like structures which collect and accentuate light around the body. The greater *chakras* lie at the outer edge of the body's aura, whereas the lesser *chakras* are positioned at its inner boundary. Each *chakra* is associated with a specific aura colour.

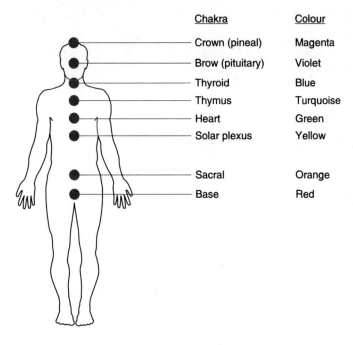

Chakra	Colour
Crown (pineal)	Magenta
Brow (pituitary)	Violet
Thyroid	Blue
Thymus	Turquoise
Heart	Green
Solar plexus	Yellow
Sacral	Orange
Base	Red

Figure 7.1 The chakras

Colour reflection reading
Patients make a choice of three colours out of eight. The three are placed in order of preference and the choice is analysed. For example, green as first choice indicates a neat and efficient person with an affinity for nature, whereas red indicates a creator and initiator, an active person.

Luscher test
Eight colours are listed in order of preference. The pattern gives an insight into the subconscious and physiological state of the patient.

Treatment
A combination of therapies is used:

coloured lights
coloured shapes
colour visualization

colour breathing – deep breathing exercises in a room with coloured light
coloured bath – delivers light refracted through water
massage with coloured oils
coloured crystals
coloured clothes and foods.

WHICH CONDITIONS ARE SUITABLE FOR TREATMENT BY COLOUR THERAPY?

- Rheumatism
- Insomnia
- Migraine
- Depression
- Asthma
- Eczema
- High blood pressure (as an adjunct to conventional medical treatment)
- Low blood pressure
- Stress, anxiety
- Post-viral fatigue syndrome
- Seasonal affective disorder
- HIV infection and AIDS (as an adjunct to conventional medical treatment)

WHICH CONDITIONS ARE NOT SUITABLE FOR TREATMENT BY COLOUR THERAPY?

- Any condition that may be caused by serious underlying disease
- Serious infections
- Epilepsy

Advantages

- Safe.
- Non-invasive.

Disadvantages

- Time and cost may be prohibitive.
- Few practitioners in the UK.

How long and how much?

First session: up to 1 hour.
Subsequent sessions: 30 minutes to 1 hour.
How many sessions? Ten to twelve.
Cost: £20–30 per session (1996 UK prices).

NHS or private? (applies to the UK only)

Colour therapy is not available on the NHS.

Simple self-help measures

- Tired and lethargic? Wear bright colours.
- Fed up, bored at work? Put an orange object on the desk
- Worried about someone or something? Visualize them or it bathed in blue light.
- Practise visualization meditation and place particular emphasis on a favourite or chosen 'healing' colour.

Addresses for referral

British Complementary Medicine
Association
9 Soar Lane
Leicester LE3 5DE
Tel. 01162 425406

Institute for Complementary Medicine
Box 194
London SE16 1QZ
Tel. 0171 237 5165

International Association of Colour
Therapists
Brook House
Avening
Tetbury
Glos GL8 8NS
Tel. 01453 832150

**Addresses for education
and training**

Institute for Complementary Medicine
(Address above)

International Association of Colour
Therapists
(Address above)

Living Colour
33 Lancaster Grove
London NW3 4EX
Tel. 0181 883 4988

8

Diagnostic aids

Iridology

Background

Iridology or *ophthalmic somatology* is a diagnostic method involving the detailed examination of the condition, colouring and markings of the iris.

Although Hippocrates mentions eye markings in his writings, the title of 'father of iridology' goes to the nineteenth-century Hungarian doctor Ignatz von Peczely. As a boy Peczely noticed a discolouration of the iris in an owl that had broken its leg. As the owl recovered the defect resolved. Many years later, as a physician, Peczely went on to publish his research and first eye charts in 1881. His work, however, was largely ignored until the 1950s when an American physician, Dr Bernard Jensen, took up his theories and re-designed the original maps to something more workable. Figure 8.1 shows a simplified version of the iridology maps that therapists use.

Iridology is often used as an aid to diagnosis by other complementary practitioners, particularly herbalists and naturopaths. It is believed that changes can occur in the iris long before an illness can manifest itself. By detecting and analysing the causes of these early changes the therapist can recommend appropriate early therapeutic measures together with changes in lifestyle and diet to maintain a sound state of health.

Research

Much evidence on the benefits of iridology has been anecdotal.

- Simon, A., Worthen, D. and Mitas, J. (1979). An evaluation of iridology. *Journal of the American Medical Association*, **242**: 1385–9.

Iridologists were shown photographs of 143 irises without meeting the patients. They did no better than chance at making a diagnosis.

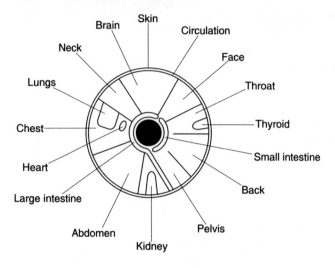

Figure 8.1 Iris map (left eye)

Mechanism of action

Changes in iris markings have been explained by the embryological connection of the eye with the central nervous system. The first sign of the developing eye appears in the 22-day-old embryo as a pair of grooves on each side of the forebrain. Eventually these outgrowths give rise to the optic nerve, retina, ciliary body (the muscle that controls the pupil diameter) and the iris. The iris may therefore receive impulses about the body's state of health from the brain. This information is then interpreted as a series of markings on the surface of the iris.

Iridologists believe that there are 28 000 nerve fibres in the iris – far more than would be required to change the size of the pupil. These fibres may carry direct messages from different organs and tissues of the body and induce change in the iris when that particular organ or tissue is affected by disease.

The techniques

A full medical history is taken including symptoms, signs, past medical history, medication, allergies, emotional functions, and social and family history. Some therapists will also carry out other tests such as urine and hair analysis.

Different iridologists will examine the irides in different ways. The most commonly used methods are:

torch and magnifying glass
slit-lamp (a tool usually used by opticians)
iris camera
video camera.

Cameras allow a record of the iris to be kept and changes compared and shown to the patient.

What does the iridologist look for?

- **Iris colour:** each colour and shade will shed light on the person's strengths and weaknesses, for example blue eyes reveal a tendency for rheumatism, whereas brown eyes indicate the person is prone to gastric problems.
- **Discolourations:** these give an indication of the state of the internal tissues, for example yellow means a chronic condition, red a build-up of iron.
- **Iris basic structure:** most therapists use comparisons with cloth (silk, net, linen and hessian). These structural types of irises also indicate personality types:
  a silk iris (tightly woven fibres) personality is a strong-willed, no-nonsense type
  a hessian iris (looser fibres) personality is easy-going and intelligent
  a net iris (like a spider's web, with large cavities) personality is non-complaining, stubborn, complex
  a linen iris (looser and more wavy fibres than silk) personality is sensitive, vulnerable and a good team-worker.
- **Detailed iris structure:** presence and position of transverse fibres (may indicate scarring, surgery), raised fibres (may indicate infection, rheumatism) and lacunae ('holes' in the iris indicating the state of a particular organ depending on their location on the iris).

Therapists cannot make a definitive diagnosis from the examination; instead, they may detect, for example a 'weakness in the immune system' which may indicate post-viral fatigue syndrome or myalgic encephalitis (ME).

Once the examination is complete a remedial or preventative programme can be discussed to address the likely conditions causing the iris markings. Most iridologists are also herbalists, naturopaths, nutritionists or homoeopaths. The therapist therefore may recommend specific treatments (e.g. reflexology, aromatherapy, acupuncture) together with lifestyle and dietary changes.

The iridologist will regularly check the patient's iris to monitor progress of treatment.

WHICH CONDITIONS ARE SUITABLE FOR TREATMENT BY IRIDOLOGY?

- Iridology is a diagnostic aid. Any condition may be seen by a practitioner

WHICH CONDITIONS ARE NOT SUITABLE FOR TREATMENT BY IRIDOLOGY?

- Any serious condition that may be caused by underlying disease. An iridologist may detect this and refer the patient to his or her general practitioner. It is more advisable for the patient to see the GP **first** to rule out any serious disease
- Serious infections

Advantages

- Safe.
- Non-invasive.
- Increasing in popularity with the general public.

Disadvantages

- Bright light may be irritable to those with sensitive eyes.
- Contact lens wearers may have iris changes from lens wear and not 'internal imbalance'.
- Time and cost may be prohibitive.
- Controversial. Many orthodox and complementary practitioners put iridology in the same class as palmistry.

How long and how much?

First session: 30 minutes to 2 hours.
Subsequent sessions: 15–30 minutes.
How many sessions? One to two to make the diagnosis, then regular sessions (one to six monthly) for follow-up.
Cost: £25–40 (1996 UK prices).

NHS or private? (applies to the UK only)

- **NHS:** not available on the NHS.
- **Private:** widely available in alternative clinics. Refer only to members of professional bodies. Most iridologists also practise other forms of complementary therapy.

Addresses for referral

British Complementary Medicine
Association
9 Soar Lane
Leicester LE3 5DE
Tel. 01162 425406

Institute for Complementary Medicine
PO Box 194
London SE16 1QZ
Tel. 0171 237 5165

National Council and Register of
Iridology
40 Stokewood Road
Swinton
Bournemouth BH3 7NC

**Addresses for education
and training**

Institute for Complementary Medicine
(Address above)

National Council and Register of
Iridology
(Address above)

Kirlian photography

Background

The basis of many complementary philosophies is that there is often a disturbance or imbalance of the vital energy flow (*chi, prana* or *shen*) which causes physical disease. Kirlian photography is a system of radiography that claims to be able to record this energy flow which appears as an aura around the body. The technique was discovered by Semyon and Valentina Kirlian, a Russian husband and wife team of radiologists.

A part of the body, most often the hand, is placed onto a highly charged photographic plate. Once developed, the photographs show a 'halo' of the hand created by the electrical interaction of the charged plate and the body's energy. It was claimed that changes in the photographs could detect changes in energy flow that *pre-empt* the onset of ill-health.

Research

No controlled studies have been undertaken into this diagnostic technique.

Mechanism of action

Interaction and interference of two energies, one from a charged plate and the other from the body, produce a 'photograph' that can be used to record and monitor the vitality of an individual.

The techniques

The hand is most commonly used. It is held on a charged plate over reactive paper. Once developed, the 'electrophotograph' indicates weaknesses in energy flow. The practitioner (who will probably practise other forms of complementary medicine) may recommend (for example) acupuncture, homoeopathy, exercise and dietary changes to strengthen this weak flow.

Regular photographs are taken to monitor progress.

WHICH CONDITIONS ARE SUITABLE FOR TREATMENT BY KIRLIAN PHOTOGRAPHY?

- Kirlian photography is a diagnostic aid. Any condition may be seen by a practitioner

WHICH CONDITIONS ARE NOT SUITABLE FOR TREATMENT BY KIRLIAN PHOTOGRAPHY?

- Any serious condition that may be caused by underlying disease. It is advisable for patients to see their GPs **first** to rule out any serious conditions

Advantages

- Non-invasive.

Disadvantages

- Unreliable: the photographic image is dependent on body temperature and pressure applied on the charged plate.

- Expensive equipment.
- Few complementary practitioners use this technique.
- Time and cost may be prohibitive for the patient.
- Controversial. Many complementary practitioners feel that it does not have enough credibility.

How long and how much?

Used by practitioners as a diagnostic aid. Cost will be included in the overall fees of the therapist.

NHS or private (applies to the UK only)

Not available on the NHS.

Addresses for referral

Contact individual complementary therapists to find out if Kirlian photography is a part of their technique.

British Complementary Medicine
Association
9 Soar Lane
Leicester LE3 5DE
Tel. 01162 425406

Institute for Complementary Medicine
PO Box 194
London SE16 1QZ
Tel. 0171 237 5165

**Address for education
and training**

Institute for Complementary Medicine
(Address above)

Radionics

Background

Radionics (or radiesthesia) is a system of diagnosis and treatment by directing 'healing energies' through special instruments to the patient *at a distance*. Radionics originated with the work of Dr Albert Abrams at Stanford University Medical College, California, in the early 1900s. Abrams accidently discovered that the note elicited from a patient's abdomen on percussion with a finger depended on the illness and the patient's alignment with the earth's electromagnetic field. Working on these findings he devised instruments that could, when attached to a patient with a specific illness, give an indication of the change in the patient's own 'energy field' measured in units of resistance (ohms).

The next big leap for radionics was in the 1930s. Ruth Drown, a Hollywood chiropractor, discovered that it was not necessary for the patient to be present or even to have met the practitioner for diagnosis or treatment. She believed that healing powers could be directed along a natural energy force that connected practitioner to patient. The instruments, often containing a lock of hair or a drop of blood, would create a link between the two. Like Eastern philosophical teachings, radionic theory accepts that all living things are surrounded and embraced by an aura of 'living energy'. Physical and psychological disease are caused by a disturbance in this energy. Practitioners believe that making a diagnosis by radionics automatically sets into motion healing energies that often start working even before a formal plan of treatment has begun.

Psionic medicine uses the same principles as radionics. It is practised by doctors using a combination of dowsing and 'miasm theory' (the presence of factors within the body that have a disruptive effect on self-healing) for diagnosis and homoeopathy for treatment.

Research

Much has been written but no controlled radionic studies have been done.

Mechanism of action

Pure thought may itself be an initiator of treatment therefore distance is irrelevant.

The input of healing energies from the practitioner via a radionic instrument re-balances the patient's spiritual, mental and physical energies.

The techniques

Diagnoses are often carried out by post, fax or telephone if the patient and practitioner are unable to meet. The practitioner remains in constant touch with the patient and provides regular feedback.

The patient is asked to complete and return a general health questionnaire and a history of the ailment. A lock of hair (the patient's 'witness') is also usually requested.

The practitioner sets up the radionic instrument (a box with a set of dials with varying calibrations and a plate to place the hair). Each symptom has a specific predetermined dial value on the instrument. The dials are adjusted according to the patient's symptoms. The practitioner 'tunes in' to the patient and tries to visualize the patient mentally. Dowsing with a pendulum is often used to find answers to simple yes/no questions the practitioner will pose. Dowsing helps to determine not only the affected organs and systems in the body but also any causative agents such as allergies, toxins and emotions.

Many practitioners will also assess the state of the *chakras* – centres in the body that act as foci of energy flow (see Figure 7.1).

Once a diagnosis has been made a treatment plan is instigated. Energy from homoeopathic remedies may be transmitted to the patient via the instrument and witness. Cards with treatment symbols or different colours may be placed on the instrument and their healing energies transmitted. Acupuncture, homoeopathy, naturopathy, etc. may also be recommended together with this therapy.

WHICH CONDITIONS ARE SUITABLE FOR TREATMENT BY RADIONICS?

- Any condition may be seen by a radionic practitioner

- Particularly useful as an adjunct
  to conventional medicine in: terminal disease
                                   dentistry

- Psychological: stress
                    anxiety
                    panic attacks

- Veterinary treatment: often a good response; some
                           practitioners only treat animals

WHICH CONDITIONS ARE NOT SUITABLE FOR TREATMENT BY RADIONICS?

- Any condition that may be caused by serious underlying disease. Although radionics is very safe, it is best to consult a general practitioner (to exclude serious problems) before embarking on a course of radionic therapy
- Serious infections

Advantages

- Very safe.
- Non-invasive.
- Easily available in the UK.

Disadvantages

- A large element of controversy in its techniques and mechanism of action.

How long and how much?

First session: 1 hour.
Subsequent sessions: 45 minutes to 1 hour.
How many sessions? Occasionally only one is required; regular follow-up is recommended to monitor the ailment.
Cost: £30–40 per session (1996 UK prices).

NHS or private? (applies to the UK only)

- **NHS:** psionic medicine is practised by doctors. This is usually available privately only. However, some GPs may combine it with their orthodox clinical practice.
- **Private:** refer only to members of professional bodies.

Addresses for referral

British Complementary Medicine
Association
9 Soar Lane
Leicester LE3 5DE
Tel. 01162 425406

Institute for Complementary Medicine
PO Box 194
London SE16 1QZ
Tel. 0171 237 5165

Psionic Medical Society
Garden Cottage
Beacon Hill Park
Hindhead
Surrey
(Doctors and dentists only)

Radionic Association Ltd
16A North Bar
Banbury
Oxford OX16 0TF
Tel. 01869 338852

Addresses for education and training

Institute for Complementary Medicine
(Address above)

Keys College of Radionics
Sycamore Farm
Chadlington
Oxford

Psionic Medical Society
(Address above; doctors and dentists
only)

9

Other therapies

Anthroposophical medicine

Anthroposophical medicine is based on the work of Rudolf Steiner (1861–1925). It is designed to be an adjunct to conventional medicine, *not* an alternative.

This therapy encourages exploration of inner feelings, intuition, emotions, instinct and spirituality. Illness, disease and accidents may have inner meaning and purpose. Some practitioners may therefore allow a symptom or disease process to continue longer than in conventional medicine to allow a more permanent recovery.

Diagnosis includes standard medical history, physical examination, laboratory tests and X-rays, as well as detailed questions on personality type, social behaviour, hobbies, etc.

- Treatments:
    homoeopathic medicines (plant, mineral or animal)
    hydrotherapy
    diets
    massage
    speech
    art therapy – painting, music, drawing, modelling (e.g. with clay), sculpture
    eurhythmy (see below)
    any conventional medical or surgical treatment.
- Used mostly in Germany, Switzerland and the Netherlands with the establishment of some hospitals that fully recognize and integrate anthroposophical and conventional medicine. In the UK inpatient treatment is available at:

    Park Attwood
    Trimpley
    Nr Bewdley
    Gloucestershire
    Tel. 01299 861444

- Courses are only open to medically qualified personnel. Any condition can therefore be treated.

Address for referral and training

Anthroposophical Medical Association
c/o Rudolph Steiner House
35 Park Road
London NW1 6XT
0171 723 4400

Bates method of eye-testing

In 1919 ophthalmologist Dr William Bates published his theories in his now famous book *Better Eyesight Without Glasses*. Believing that poor eyesight may be due to tension and poor function and development in ocular muscles that help focusing, Bates developed a system of re-training by general relaxation and specfic exercises for the eye muscles. These exercises involve:

- Palming: cover the eyes with the hands to shut out all light.
- Near/far focusing: focus alternately on near and far objects.
- Swinging: swing the head and body smoothly to and fro, the eyes are focused in the distance but move with the head.
- Blinking: a few minutes of rapid blinking, three or four times daily.

Bates' most famous success was Aldous Huxley who was restored to full sight from near-blindness.

The method is useful for myopia (short sight), hypermetropia (long sight), squint and astigmatism.

Few practitioners are available in the UK.

Address for referral and training

The Bates Association
PO Box 25
Shoreham by Sea
Sussex BN43 6ZF
Tel. 01273 881190

Biochemic tissue salts

Biochemic tissue salts were developed in the late 1900s by the German homoeopath Dr Wilhelm Schuessler.

Extracted from plant material, 12 salts (e.g. sodium chloride, magnesium phosphate, calcium fluoride) were originally used by Schuessler to replace deficiencies and correct mineral imbalances within the body.

Tissue salts are dispensed in a lactose tablet and are available from larger chemists and homoeopathic pharmacists. They are safe to use at home for minor ailments.

Bowen technique

The Bowen technique is a gentle, subtle form of massage originating in Australia. Therapists also advise on home remedies for certain ailments.

The technique is suitable for musculoskeletal problems (e.g. back pain) and sports injuries.

For referral, contact local complementary medicine clinics.

Colonic irrigation

Colonic irrigation is a method of washing out the lower colon and rectum with warm water. Practitioners believe that irrigation stops toxin build-up and helps prevent disease. The technique has enjoyed recent popularity with many public figures endorsing its benefits.

It is dangerous in patients with bowel problems, e.g. Crohn's disease, ulcerative colitis, rectal bleeding.

- Cost: £30–40 per session (1996 UK prices).
- Available in health clinics and some natural therapy centres.

Address for information

Colonic International Association
16 Englands Lane
London NW3 4TG
Tel. 0171 483 1595

Conductive education

Conductive education was first developed in Hungary in 1945 by Andras Peto. It is a system of special education for children and adults with motor disorders.

The aims of the therapy are to improve motor skills and function and positively affect the emotional and intellectual abilities of the patient. Professional teachers are called 'conductors' and are responsible for the physical, intellectual, social and personal development of the patient. Initial training takes four years. Conductive education is given in groups and one-to-one teaching with particular emphasis on drill and rhythm.

The main publicity for conductive education came after 1986 when British children suffering from cerebral palsy were given full-time help at the Peto Institute, Budapest, with impressive results.

Motor problems suitable for 'treatment' include cerebral palsy and spina bifida in children, and Parkinson's disease, multiple sclerosis, strokes and head injuries in adults.

Address for referral and training

Birmingham Institute for Conductive Education
Bell Hill
Northfield
Birmingham B31 1LD
Tel. 0121 477 0801

The institute offers group work and individual consultation, as well as private treatment for children (up to 11 years old) and adults. Residential education is also available. There is a monthly newsletter, *Conduct!*

Crystal and gem therapy

Crystals and gemstones have certain vibrational characteristics which can aid in healing certain ailments. Practitioners believe that crystals are transformers of energy and that they are able to focus and balance energies. The increasing use of crystals in technology (e.g. radio technology, computers and watches) has focused attention on this type of therapy.

Most stones are worn close to the body, kept in the home, in the car, etc. Occasionally the stones are steeped in water and the resulting lotion used to treat disease. In ancient times crystals and gems were crushed and used as a lotion for wounds and an antidote for poison.

Clients pick a stone from a selection according to their ailment, personality, plans for the future, etc. Examples are:

- Moonstone: protection for travellers; treatment of fevers; 'stimulator' of the mind.

- Turquoise: treatment of poor eyesight, inflammation, protector of horses and riders.
- Diamond: protection against disease.
- Amber (not actually a stone but solidified resin): disinfectant; treatment for fevers, asthma, hay fever, catarrh and chest infections.

Crystal therapy is often used as an adjunct to other therapies, especially colour and sound therapy.

Electrocrystal therapy uses crystals to amplify electromagnetic waves which are then directed at the patient. The pattern produced when these waves interfere with the body's energies are used to identify the location of energy imbalance. Once a diagnosis has been made this imbalance is redressed by exposure to certain vibrational frequencies.

Addresses for information and referral

British Complementary Medicine
Association
9 Soar Lane
Leicester LE3 5DE
Tel. 01162 425406

Institute of Crystal and Gem Therapists
2 Kerswell Cottages
Exeter
Devon
Tel. 01392 832669

Mr H. Oldfield
Electro-Crystal Therapy
117 Long Drive
South Ruislip
Midx HA4 0HG
Tel. 0181 841 1716

Enzyme-potentiated desensitization

Hyposensitization of patients from their allergies (e.g. hay fever, rhinitis, eczema) is achieved by the use of small doses of allergens. Typically, treatment is 9–12 injections over 2–3 years with occasional top-up doses.

This can be a **dangerous** practice. Refer **only** to an experienced medical practitioner.

Address for referral

Royal London Homoeopathic Hospital
NHS Trust
Great Ormond Street
London WC1N 3HR
Tel. 0171 837 8833

Eurhythmy

Eurhythmy is a system of therapy through physical movement to music, created by Rudolf Steiner as a part of anthroposophical medicine. Postures, gentle movement and dance steps are linked to certain vowels, consonants and vocalizations.

The aim of therapy is to improve posture and function, encourage relaxation, improve breath control, alter emotional responses, help concentration, etc. Therapy is often given in conjunction with other anthroposophical treatments.

For referral and training, see 'Anthroposophical medicine, above.

Facial diagnosis

Facial diagnosis originated in traditional Chinese medicine and concepts of *chi* and the balance of *yin* and *yang* (see Chapter 2).

The face is divided into zones that correspond with the body systems and internal organs (Figure 9.1). Changes in marking, texture and colour indicate state of health. Symmetry, size, shape and positioning of the facial features indicate intellect, personality and constitutional type.

- Eyebrows: thick eyebrows indicate a strong character; brows meeting in the middle show intelligence.
- Ears: high-set ears indicate intelligence.
- Lower lip: a swollen lip suggests a sluggish bowel, constipation.

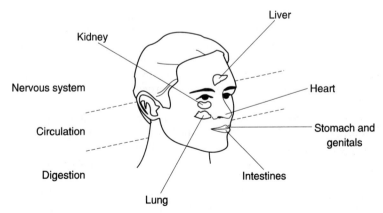

Figure 9.1 Facial diagnosis

Flotation therapy

Flotation therapy is a form of sensory deprivation achieved by lying in a dark, warm, soundless tank of saline about 25 cm deep. The concentration of saline allows the body to float freely. It is used for stress relief, relaxation and as an aid to visualization therapy and autogenics.

* Problems:
    not suitable for those with a nervous disposition or claustrophobia
    hygiene – water is often not changed after each patient.
* Available at health clinics, natural health clinics and specialist flotation centres.
* Cost: 1 hour float – £20–30 (1996 UK prices).

Address for information

Flotation Tank Association
PO Box 11024
London SW4 7ZF
Tel. 0171 627 4962

Healing

The term 'healing' includes *faith healing* and *spiritual healing*. Faith healing depends upon the patients' belief of self-cure. Suggestion and placebo effects play a central role.

Spiritual healers transmit energy from themselves to the patient or act as a channel for a 'universal life force'. After a gesture or ritual the healer may place a hand on or near the patient's head. The patient is asked to relax and concentrate on breathing, inner warmth and light. Sessions last for about an hour with weekly treatments. Therapists aim to re-balance energies with a *gradual* return to health.

Absent healing or healing from afar is practised if the patient cannot get to the healer owing to ill-health or distance.

Faith is not a prerequisite for treatment. Some healers have worked successfully on animals. Most professional spiritual healers do not have religious links.

Healing can be used for disease prevention and health promotion but is particularly good for the relief of pain and distress, especially in terminally ill patients.

Addresses for referral

Association of Therapeutic Healers
Flat 5
54–56 Neal Street
London WC2 9PA
Tel. 0171 240 0176

National Federation of Spiritual Healers
Old Manor Farm Studio
Church Street
Sunbury on Thames
Midx TW16 6RG
Tel. 01932 783164

British Alliance of Healing Associations
23 Nutcroft Grove
Fetcham
Leatherhead
Surrey KT22 9LD
Tel. 01372 373241

Address for training

College of Healing
Runnings Park
Croft Bank
West Malvern
Worcs WR12 4BP
Tel. 01684 566450

Hydrotherapy

Hydrotherapy is the use of water for special treatments – Jacuzzi, spas, aerated pools, steam baths, sitz baths (alternate hot and cold bathing), inhalations and drinking (mineral waters).

Water births are now in vogue. The mother gives birth while standing or sitting in a large birthing pool. Advocates claim less painful childbirth and less distress to the child. Hydrotherapy to help ease labour pains is also increasing. The woman is more mobile and the feel and warmth of the water can encourage relaxation. There is less pressure on the abdomen which probably allows more circulation to the uterine muscles and subsequently less pain.

The most common use in conventional medicine is as an aid to physiotherapy. Patients carry out exercises in water, the buoyancy of the water lifting body weight off inflamed, painful or damaged joints. It is particularly useful for arthritis and sports injuries.

Some sufferers of myalgic encephalomyelitis (ME) or post-viral fatigue syndrome have found that daily cold baths and showers help symptoms.

In complementary medicine hydrotherapy is used by many different disciplines, especially naturopaths.

Address for referral and training

UK College of Hydrotherapy
515 Hagley Road
Bearwood
Birmingham B66 4AX
Tel. 0121 429 9191
(See also under 'Naturopathy')

Integration therapy

Integration therapy is based on the premise that certain ailments are caused by the persistence of neonatal reflexes into adulthood. The individual then responds abnormally to given situations causing physiological and psychological stresses.

Examination and diagnosis of abnormal reflexes by a therapist is followed by an exercise regimen to introduce adult reflexes into the patient's lifestyle.

This therapy is suitable for musculoskeletal ailments (back pain, muscular aches), psychological problems (phobias, anxiety) and childhood developmental and behavioural problems.

By their very nature reflexes will take time to be 'taught out' or 'taught into' the system. Therapy therefore tends to be prolonged (18 months to 2 years) and expensive.

Address for information and referral

Institute for Developmental Potential
6 Patna Place
North Road West
Plymouth
Devon PL1 5AY
Tel. 01752 222188

Iscador therapy

Iscador is a mistletoe extract used by anthroposophical doctors and homoeopaths. Its main use is as an adjunct to conventional therapy for malignant disease. Iscador helps in control of symptoms such as pain, nausea and vomiting, and improves the patient's quality of life.

Iscador can be taken by mouth or by injection. The mechanism of action is probably through stimulation of the immune system.

Address for referral

Royal London Homoeopathic Hospital
NHS Trust
Great Ormond Street
London WC1N 3HR
Tel. 0171 837 8833

Jin shin jyutsu

A Japanese system of touch, gentle massage and exercises helps clear congestion in 'energy locks' and allow the free flow of internal energy or *chi*. It is suitable as a method of health maintenance as well as disease management. Patients with post-viral fatigue syndrome (ME) may benefit particularly.

Address for information and referral

Southsea Centre for Complementary Medicine
25 Osborne Road
Southsea
Hants PO5 3ND
Tel. 01705 874748

Magnetotherapy

A system of therapy using magnets and their electromagnetic fields, magnetotherapy first gained publicity when astronauts were treated for 'space sickness' using magnetism. Nausea, lethargy and generalized debility were caused by time out of the earth's electromagnetic field. Recreating an artificial field around the astronauts by magnets fixed into their space suits solved the problem.

Individuals in large towns and cities may be suffering from under-exposure to the earth's electromagnetic field caused by interference from the trappings of modern urbanization. Magnetotherapy works by affecting the flow of positively and negatively charged particles in the tissues, fluid spaces and blood. Research indicates that magnetism can positively affect tissue and wound healing processes.

Magnetotherapy is indicated for musculoskeletal injuries and arthritis. Therapists also claim increased vitality and general well-being. Some therapists may apply magnets to acupuncture points in musculoskeletal disorders. Patients are able to buy shoes, garments and furniture that contain magnets to allow 24-hour exposure.

This therapy is *not* suitable for patients with pacemakers or cochlear implants.

Address for information and referral

The Hale Clinic
7 Park Crescent
London W1V 3HE
Tel. 0171 631 0156/637 3377

Manual lymphatic drainage

Manual lymphatic drainge originated in France in the 1930s; it is a form of massage to stimulate active flow of lymph, helping to eliminate toxins and excess fluid. Therapists can help patients with swollen ankles, cellulite, puffy eyes, bloated abdomens and generalized fluid retention.

Patients with fluid retention secondary to heart disease (congestive cardiac failure) or cancer need to consult their doctor before undergoing this therapy.

Patients with lymphoedema (swollen limb due to a blockage in lymph flow – usually secondary to cancerous spread) are being increasingly helped with gentle massage by trained nurses on cancer wards. This not only increases patient comfort but also promotes a therapeutic relationship between nurse and patient.

- Cost: £30 for a 1-hour session (1996 UK prices).

Address for information and referral

MLD UK
8 Wittenham Lane
Dorchester on Thames
Oxon OX10 7JW

Neurolinguistic programming

Neurolinguistic programming (NLP) developed in the 1970s out of the ideas and practices of three leading psychotherapists (Milton Erickson, Virginia Satir and Fritz Perls) to bring about significant change in human behaviour.

- Why NLP?
    'neuro' – neurological processes of the five senses used to experience the environment and develop behaviour

'linguistic' – language for communication to others and the self (thought)
'programming' – individuals programme their thoughts, ideas and behaviours.

- NLP is concerned with how successful people achieve their success and how their thought processes and behaviour patterns can be copied and 'programmed' into others.

Essentials of NLP

- Maps: each person has a different 'mental map' of their experiences and thoughts which is reflected in their behaviour. Understanding and appreciating the differences in each individual's mental map allows for better communication and relationships.
- Intention: behaviour has a positive intention (whether it is conscious or subconscious). By finding other ways to achieve this positive intention an individual can change unwanted behaviours.
- Communication: successful communication is judged by the results it achieves. If results are unsatisfactory, change the ways and method of communication.
- Failure is feedback: use the feedback of 'failure' as a positive learning tool and a way to change behaviour.
- Options: the more the better.
- Flexibility: the more flexible one's behaviour, the more influence one has.

Applications

Neurolinguistic programming is very popular in the USA and increasingly so in the UK, particularly in the fields of personal development, business, education and sport. It is also useful as a therapeutic tool for:

phobias
stress
depression
smoking
eating disorders
nail-biting
chronic pain
post-viral fatigue syndrome or ME.

The main advantage of this therapy is that it is not practitioner-dependent. Patients can learn techniques and apply them in every-day situations.

- **Self-help:** to treat stress (e.g. in a traffic jam, at work, etc.) – think of a favourite picture or scene; try to visualize every detail, using all your senses. Then press on your first knuckle; the visual picture is now associated with pressure or a tap on this knuckle. The second, third and fourth knuckles can similarly be allocated to other pictures, music or sensations. Next time you are stressed, press on a knuckle and the picture or thoughts will automatically appear. With practice this becomes an extremely effective technique.

Address for information

Association of NLP
48 Corser Street
Old Swinford
Stourbridge
W. Midlands PY8 2DQ
Tel. 01384 443935

Pilates method

Developed by Joseph Pilates in America in the early 1900s, this method is particularly good for 'bad backs'. A series of exercises and postures help to strengthen abdominal, lateral and back muscles, developing a strong 'central body core' which acts like 'scaffolding'.

- Cost: £20–25 per session or class (1996 UK prices).

Address for referral

Association of Pilates Teachers
Body Control Studios
17 Queensberry Mews West
London SW7 2DY
Tel. 0171 581 7041

Probiotics

Probiotics is the use of supplements of 'friendly' bacteria such as lactobacilli and bifidobacteria, which also occur naturally in the intestinal tract, to improve nutrition and protect against disease.

Advocates of therapy believe that probiotic bacteria are particularly effective against bacterial, fungal and viral infections of the kidney, bladder, vagina and gastrointestinal tract. They may also have anticarcinogenic effects, as well as helping to reduce cholesterol and improve liver function.

Supplements need to contain several billion live, viable organisms per gram and must be kept refrigerated. Powdered products contain many more viable organisms. Liquids tend to be unstable and often contain no living organisms.

- Supplements should be taken 1 hour before meals with water.
- Probiotic therapy is safe in children and pregnant women.

Radiance technique (Reiki)

The basic concept of radiance technique is a lack of 'universal energy' in the patient. The technique originated from the Far East in ancient Sanskrit *sutras* (writings). Radiance technique teachers can take up to 16 years to learn the 'seven degrees' of therapy, which has been found useful to enhance quality of life in many chronic conditions such as cancer, AIDS and post-viral fatigue syndrome.

Gentle touch, manipulation, pressure techniques, dietary manipulation and exercises allow universal energy back into the patient. Energy exchange between patient and practitioner helps the therapeutic process.

**Addresses for information
and referral**

Radiance Education Unlimited
9 Finedon Hall
Finedon
Northants NN9 5NL
Tel. 01933 681900

Reiki Alliance
27 Lavington Road
Ealing
London W13 9NN
Tel. 0181 579 3813

T'ai chi ch'uan

T'ai chi ch'uan is a Chinese exercise, not a martial art, that dates back over six centuries to the Buddhists. It is still widely practised today in China, typically at early morning sessions in parks.

The basic form has 40 movements. The more complex form has over a hundred. These simple, slow, graceful movements are particularly useful for general exercise, relaxation, contemplation, relief of muscular aches and pains, stress and health promotion.

Address for information

British T'ai Chi Ch'uan Association and London T'ai Chi Academy
7 Upper Wimpole Street
London W1M 7TD
Tel. 0171 935 8444

Tea tree oil

The tea tree (*Melaleuca alternifolia*) grows only in Australia. Its oil has been found to have antibacterial and antifungal properties, and is useful in the treatment of acne, bites, burns and skin infections.

- Available in several forms for use in massage, bathing, and anti-septic wipes.
- Cost:
    aromatherapy oil £4.15 for 10 ml
    cream £3.50 for 100 g (1996 UK prices).

Zero balancing

Zero balancing is a relatively new therapy based on osteopathic techniques and Chinese theories of energy flow. Therapy aims to ease muscle and joint problems by manipulation and the re-balance of internal energy flow. It works well for musculoskeletal disorders (e.g. back and neck pains) and stress.

- Cost: £25–35 per session (1996 UK prices).

Address for information and referral

Zero Balance Association UK
36 Richmond Road
Cambridge CB4 3PU
Tel. 01223 315480

Zinc therapy

Zinc is important in wound healing, fertility, and in DNA and protein synthesis. It is also essential in several cell biochemical processes. A deficiency results in poor resistance to infection, a reduced sense of taste and dry skin.

Some health shops have a 'taste test' to check zinc levels.

- Zinc lozenges may shorten the duration of colds.
- Zinc-based creams (e.g. zinc oxide or zinc castor) are useful for infective rashes, dermatitis and nappy rash.

Oysters are the richest source of zinc available. Other rich sources include wholemeal bread and pasta, brown rice, and whole grains and nuts.

Part Two

Common conditions and their treatment

10

Complementary therapies for common conditions

Anxiety

What is it?

Anxiety is an over-reaction to good or bad, emotional or physical stressful situations, such as marriage, divorce, job interview, examinations or illness. Symptoms include racing heart, sweaty palms, trembling, chronic headaches, insomnia, depression, dizzy spells and muscular aches and pains. It affects 5% of the population, mainly young adults, women twice as much as men.

General anxiety is often punctuated by bouts of acute anxiety or panic attacks.

Cause

Anxiety is caused by an abnormal reaction to everyday situations and stress causing excessive adrenaline production (the 'fight or flight' reaction).

Self-help

- Listen to relaxation tapes and learn simple relaxation and meditation techniques.
- Stretch and massage affected muscles.
- Avoid stimulants such as coffee, tea, nicotine and alcohol.
- Take regular exercise to 'burn off' the excess adrenaline.

Conventional treatment

Counselling
Many general practitioners now employ counsellors in their surgeries. *Insight psychotherapy* (to uncover unconscious conflicts) and *supportive psychotherapy* (to reduce symptoms) may help in selected patients.

Drug therapy
Beta-blockers can help symptoms – short-term use only (*not* in asthmatic patients).

Some patients may need long-term antidepressant therapy. The selective serotonin re-uptake inhibitor (SSRI), paroxetine, may be particularly helpful.

Complementary therapy

Acupuncture
Helps reduce anxiety and aids relaxation.

Acupressure
Press on points for 1–2 minutes:
    Colon 4
    Liver 3
    Heart Protector 6 (two fingerbreadths up from the wrist crease in the midline).
For point location, see Chapter 2.

Aromatherapy and massage
Oils used are sandalwood, basil, geranium and lavender.

Homoeopathy
Tarentula 6C for stress and difficulty in relaxing (every 2 hours, up to 10 doses).
    For chronic anxiety and panic attacks, seek expert advice.

Herbal medicine
Teas or infusions made from camomile or clover blossom ease the general feeling of anxiety and its symptoms.

Hypnosis
Works well with relaxation and meditation techniques.

Meditation
Transcendental meditation, yoga and zen are techniques that need to be learnt with daily practice.

Naturopathy and nutrition
Calcium, magnesium, vitamin B complex and vitamin C are often recommended together with cleansing treatments and self-help measures.

Other therapies
Many complementary therapies are useful in anxiety and stress disorders, e.g. reflexology, t'ai chi and Bach flower remedies.

Arthritis

What is it?

There are two main types of arthritis:

- **Rheumatoid arthritis** (RA) affects any age; characterized by a symmetrical swelling, inflammation, stiffness and pain of the joints. The disease can affect the whole body and systemic problems such as fatigue, anaemia and carpal tunnel syndrome can occur. Women are affected 2–3 times more commonly than men. More common in temperate climates.
- **Osteoarthritis** (OA): 'wear and tear' of the joints. Most people have a minor degree of OA by 40 years of age, and the condition is universal by age 70. Mild aches and pains are the main symptoms. The weight-bearing joints (knees and hips) are most affected.

Other less common but related types of disease include psoriatic arthritis, ankylosing spondylitis, Reiter's syndrome, Behçet's syndrome and gout.

Cause

All forms of arthritis (particularly RA) affect the synovial membrane which lines each joint and produces the lubricating synovial fluid. This helps to decrease friction and allows efficient and painless movement of joints. Inflammation of the synovial membrane and a lack of synovial fluid contribute to slow joint destruction with gradual development of symptoms.

Self-help

- Lose weight to ease burden on affected joints, especially the hips and knees.
- 'Watercise' – walking in a swimming pool at a depth where the water reaches the chest. The buoyancy of the water lifts weight off the knees and hips. Water resistance allows muscles to exercise gently.

- Cycling is a good non-weight-bearing exercise that maintains mobility and strength in muscles.
- Use ice-packs to help prevent pain: e.g. a bag of frozen peas in a damp cloth, for 15 minutes each hour.
- Use heat treatments for acute flare-ups of symptoms and pain.
- Dietary precautions: some sufferers may be helped by avoiding dairy products.

Conventional treatment

Simple analgesia (e.g. paracetamol, co-proxamol), anti-inflammatory drugs (e.g. ibuprofen, diclofenac) and physiotherapy are mainstays of treatment. Rheumatoid arthritis needs specialist treatment, especially in the younger patient. Some patients with severe arthritis may be suitable for joint replacement surgery.

Complementary therapy

Acupressure
Press on each point for 1–2 minutes:
    knee pain – Gallbladder 34
    hand pain – Colon 4
    hip pain – Gallbladder 30 (side of the buttock, over the inner hollow by the greater trochanter of the femur).
For point location see Chapter 2.

Acupuncture
Excellent for pain relief, increasing mobility and cutting down on anlgesic intake.

Naturopathy and nutrition
Fasting for 24 hours on vegetable juice (e.g. carrot, celery, tomato) once weekly may help.
    Vitamins A, B and C, and evening primrose oil may also be beneficial.

Hydrotherapy
Spas, steam baths and mud baths help ease pain. Avoid in acute attacks.

Green-lipped mussel extract
See Chapter 4.

Homoeopathy
Aconite 30C, arnica 30C, pulsatilla 6C – four times daily. Seek expert advice for severe pain and illness.

Aromatherapy and massage
These therapies complement each other well and help ease muscle stiffness and help mobility. Oils used are basil, jasmine, rosemary, marjoram and lemongrass.

Herbal medicine
Teas or infusions made from garlic, devil's claw or meadowsweet for general aches and pains; red clover for inflammation.

Chinese herbal medicine
Seek expert advice.

Other therapies
Reflexology, hypnosis and meditation will help relieve muscle tensions and pain.

Asthma

What is it?

Reversible airways narrowing and inflammation of the bronchioles (smaller airways) causing wheezing and cough (often only at night). Severe asthma causes rapid respiration, shortness of breath, a tightness in the chest and is a **medical emergency**.

Cause

- Allergies to pollen, moulds, dust, animal dander, house dust mites, foodstuffs (e.g. egg, artificial colourants, wheat, milk, nuts, seafood).
- Air pollution.
- Emotional stress.
- Non-specific viral infections (e.g. a cold). Infants under 1 year old often become wheezy with a viral infection. They are *not* necessarily asthmatic. The wheeze is due to congestion of the already narrow bronchioles.
- Hereditary – especially if other conditions are present such as eczema, hay fever, allergic rhinitis.

Self-help

- Avoid allergens, vacuum mattress (to eliminate dust mite).
- Stop smoking and avoid smoke-filled rooms.
- Avoid cold air, use a scarf and breathe through the nose.
- Take regular exercise, especially any sport requiring short bursts of activity, e.g. swimming, tennis and golf.
- Avoid aspirin or aspirin-related painkillers such as ibuprofen. Asthmatics can develop an allergy to these drugs which can make asthma worse – sometimes with fatal consequences.

Conventional treatment

- Inhaled bronchodilators (e.g. salbutamol – a reliever) and anti-inflammatory inhalers (e.g. sodium cromoglycate and beclomethasone – preventers) are the mainstays of treatment.
- The aim of therapy is to **prevent** onset of an asthmatic attack by taking regular 'preventers'. Poor inhaler technique and poor compliance are common reasons for badly controlled asthma. Many general practices now have asthma clinics run by highly trained nurses exclusively for sufferers.

Complementary therapy

It is extremely important to *continue with conventional medical treatment* while trying complementary therapy.

Acupuncture
Acupuncture has a significant short-term effect on asthma. It can help to reduce steroid (preventer) intake. Patients often need regular top-up sessions every 1–3 months.

Some Chinese clinics use acupuncture daily over prolonged periods and claim good results. Many patients find this impractical.

Acupressure
Press on points for 1–2 minutes:
    Asthma relief point (1 fingerbreadth either side of the 7th cervical vertebra (base of the neck).
    Lung 7 (see Chapter 2).

Homoeopathy
Remedies used are arsenicum and nat. mur. Homoeopathy works especially well for asthma that is triggered by a specific allergen (see above). Seek expert homoeopathic advice.

Other therapies
Since emotions can aggravate asthma, relaxation techniques may also help, such as aromatherapy, reflexology, massage and hydrotherapy. Pupils of the Alexander and Feldenkrais techniques, self-hypnosis, autogenics and biofeedback may also find help with these methods.

Back pain

What is it?

Four out of five people will have back pain at some time in their lives.

Thirty-five patients out of 1000 on a general practitioner's list present with acute low back pain in any one year.

In the community, 60% of individuals complain of back pain at some point in any 2-week period.

Most people will suffer from lower back pain ('mechanical back pain') at some stage of their lives.

Occasionally this may be accompanied by sciatica – pain and/or tingling radiating down the leg.

Cause

The spinal column consists of vertebrae, muscles, tendons and ligaments. All these structures can become sprained, strained or move out of place, causing pain.

Sciatica is caused by irritation or pressure on the main nerve of the leg. Pain radiates along the path of the nerve.

A *'slipped disc'* occurs when one of the discs between the vertebrae gets squashed and bulges forward or sideways. The symptoms are acute back pain with difficulty in moving, sciatica and occasional weakness in the ankle or foot. More rarely it can present with problems with the bowels or bladder.

Most acute back problems are due to lifting or trying to lift heavy objects. However, many people can suffer back pain from awkwardly getting out of a car, sneezing, bending, pulling, twisting, etc.

Self-help

- Rest flat for a *maximum* of 24–36 hours only. Then move around slowly and start simple exercises to loosen and stretch the muscles. Books and videos on back care, GPs or physiotherapists can advise on exercises.
- A rolled-up towel or pillow under the small of the back and knees helps provide additional support to back muscles.
- Swimming gently or walking in a pool up to chest level is beneficial – the buoyancy of the water supports the weight of the body helping to rest the back muscles; gentle exercises in the pool will be more effective.
- Ice treatment – a bag of frozen peas in a damp cloth applied for 15 minutes every hour will help to ease pain. Alternating this with heat treatment will also settle the pain.
- Heat treatment only – *after* the first 2 days of ice.

Prevention of back pain

- Exercise regularly to strengthen the back muscles.
- Reduce weight if obese.
- Take care when lifting. Always bend the knees and keep the back straight.
- Roll out of bed slowly rather than springing out.
- Improve posture at work, at home and in the car; use a firm chair in the office, an extra cushion for the car seat. Some sufferers change their cars altogether.
- Sitting for too long puts strain on the discs. Stand and walk around regularly – hourly if possible.
- Sleeping on the stomach strains back muscles. Change to sleeping on the side or back.
- Sleep on a bed with a firm mattress. A board (or old door) under a soft mattress will help. Alternatively, move the mattress to the floor. A waterbed will support all the important parts of the back and many sufferers have invested in one.
- Obtain additional information and advice from:

National Back Pain Association
16 Elmtree Road
Teddington
Midx TW11 8ST
Tel. 0181 977 5474

Conventional treatment

Simple analgesia (co-proxamol) or anti-inflammatory drugs may be prescribed. Patients with severe pain and muscle spasm may do well with 2–3 days on a muscle relaxant such as diazepam. X-rays do not affect the management of back pain and are not routinely carried out.

Physiotherapy may be arranged to help pain and mobility and educate the patient in exercises and back care. Rarely, surgery may be carried out for persistent acute pain due to a 'slipped disc' or neurological problems if conservative treatment has failed.

Complementary therapy

Osteopathy and chiropractice
These therapies involve moving various spinal structures within their normal range of movement. Two or three sessions are usually adequate. Practitioners also help with exercise advice. Patients occasionally report a dramatic recovery.

Acupuncture
Local trigger or tender points are used. Weekly sessions for 4 weeks should help pain and mobility.

Acupressure
Press on points for 1–2 minutes:
   sciatica – Bladder 60
   back pain – Bladder 23.
For point location see Chapter 2.

Aromatherapy and massage
These therapies work well together to loosen and relax tight muscles and improve range of movement. Oils used are sage, basil, lavender and rosemary.

Homoeopathy
Good as first-aid. Arnica 6X, 1 tablet 2-hourly during an acute attack is often effective.

Alexander and Feldenkrais techniques
These techniques strengthen the back and prevent or reduce acute episodes of pain.

Meditation
Visualization helps with pain control.

T'ai chi
The gentle, slow movements help exercise and strengthen back muscles.

Rolfing
Deep massage will help loosen and relax muscles. Practitioners also help with exercise advice.

Pilates method
Exercises to strengthen anterior and lateral abdominal muscles help ease back pain and are useful in prevention of chronic backache (see Chapter 9).

Behavioural problems in children

What is it?

The behavioural problem known as *attention deficit disorder* (ADD) usually presents with hyperkinesis or hyperactivity involving disturbed sleep patterns, poor attention and concentration, aggressiveness, irritability, disobedience, inability to stop talking or interrupting, fidgeting, frustration, difficulty in making friends, appetite disturbance and attention-seeking behaviour. It is much more common in boys than girls (10 : 1), and may affect up to 5% of schoolchildren.

Cause

- Child abuse: physical, emotional and sexual.
- Neurological damage: through childbirth, infection or an acquired syndrome.
- Food sensitivities: foods implicated include those containing natural salicylates, additives, colourants, dairy products, artificial sweeteners and sugar.

Self-help

- Find a teacher who is skilled with an overactive child.
- Do not *require* the child to sit still for long periods.

Conventional treatment

Behavioural and cognitive therapies are given under the care of a child psychiatrist. Parents are referred for parent training and behaviour management.

Drug treatments include antidepressants and ritalin.

Complementary therapy

Nutrition

To assess whether a child has food sensitivities parents should be instructed to eliminate all food additives, colourings and naturally occurring salicylates for 3–4 weeks (Boxes 10.1–10.3). If this is unsuccessful, eliminate milk and sugar also from the diet for another 2 weeks. If there is still no response, gradually re-introduce foods one by one and watch for a reaction. Food re-introduction can often produce a swift recurrence of acute symptoms. If food elimination methods do not work it is advisable for the GP to review the child for further assessment. In some cases specialist referral may be appropriate.

- **Supplements:** there may be a link between zinc, food intolerance and hyperactivity. Oil of evening primrose has improved the behaviour of hyperactive children, suggesting they may lack an essential fatty acid. Doses recommended:
  zinc citrate 15 mg at night
  oil of evening primrose 500 mg at night.

BOX 10.1 Foods containing high levels of salicylates – STOP

Fruit	apples, oranges, plums, pineapple, tomatoes, dried fruit, peaches, apricots, nectarines, aubergines, avocados, melons, grapefruit, grapes, cherries, lychees, berries, currants
Vegetables	canned sweetcorn, broad beans, courgettes, radishes, peppers, cucumber, watercress, asparagus
Sweets	strong mints, liquorice
Nuts	peanuts, almonds, water chestnuts
Preserves and sauces	jams, marmalade, jelly, cider vinegar
Drinks	tea, coffee, Ribena, cola, apple juice, grape juice, orange juice, pineapple juice

---

BOX 10.2 Foods containing moderate levels of salicylates – LIMIT to two portions daily

Fruit	mango, papaya, pears, rhubarb, pomegranates, lemons, limes, passion fruit
Vegetables	fresh sweetcorn, cauliflower, marrow, spinach, carrots, sweet potato, parsnips, beetroot, broccoli, potato (unpeeled), garlic, mushrooms
Nuts	walnuts, hazelnuts, brazil nuts, coconut, pistachios
Preserves and sauces	lime jam and marmalade
Drinks	lemonade, limeade

BOX 10.3 Foods containing little or no salicylates

Fruit	peeled pears, kiwi fruit, bananas
Vegetables	peeled potato (e.g. chips), cabbage, shallots, leeks, sprouts, swede, green beans, dried beans and peas, bamboo shoots, lentils parsley, lettuce, celery
Nuts	all those not listed in Boxes 10.1 and 10.2
Drinks	dandelion coffee, herb tea, Ovaltine, pear juice

Cancer

What is it?

Cell division and growth is normally under strict control. A cancer cell somehow becomes subtly different (mutates) and escapes from the body's direct control. Growth is unrestrained and the tumour ultimately exerts its effects by its size, its spread to distant organs (liver, bone, kidney, lungs, etc.) and its secretion of hormones.

Cause

Genetic susceptibility is implicated, as are external factors such as smoking, diet, environmental pollutants and ultraviolet light.

Conventional treatment

Treatment is based on surgery, radiotherapy, chemotherapy and palliative medicine. In the UK, community district and Macmillan

nurses, in addition to the patient's general practitioner and specialist, are available for support, counselling and general advice.

Complementary therapy

Naturopathy and nutrition
Many diets are aimed at *preventing* cancer and seek to eliminate
cancer-causing foods (carcinogens) from the diet. Patients suffering
from cancer should seek expert advice, but the basic dietary principles include:

- Avoid sugar and salt.
- Avoid processed foods, preservatives and colourings.
- Avoid caffeine, alcohol and tobacco.
- Reduce intake of fatty foods, e.g. red meat, cheeses, chocolate,
  fried foods.
- Increase intake of natural, unprocessed foods, e.g. brown bread,
  pasta, cereals.
- Increase intake of fresh fruit and vegetables.
- Increase intake of live yoghurt.
- Increase natural protein, e.g. chicken, eggs, fish, beans.
- Increase vitamin intake, especially vitamins A, B complex,
  C and E.
- Increasing mineral intake (iron, potassium, selenium, mag-
  nesium, copper, manganese and calcium) may also help.

Acupressure
Pressing on Colon 4 for 1–2 minutes at a time will help relaxation
and reduce anxiety. For point location see Chapter 2.

Acupuncture
Used for pain relief and reducing the side-effects of radiotherapy
and chemotherapy (e.g. nausea and vomiting).

Homoeopathy and Chinese herbal medicine
Used as an adjunct to conventional treatment to help relieve pain
and side-effects of conventional treatment. Seek expert advice.

Herbal medicine
Use teas or infusions:

chamomile, calendula, marigold – calming, relaxation
fennel, peppermint, slippery elm – bowel upsets, colic
rosemary – muscle cramps and spasm
red sage – catarrh.

Aromatherapy, massage and reflexology
Massage with aromatic oils (e.g. rosemary, cedarwood, lavender) will help reduce anxiety, muscle tension and help relaxation. The advantage of these methods is that they can be easily carried out by carers.

Meditation
Breathing exercises, visualization and imagery all help relaxation, anxiety and depression.

Iscador therapy
A mistletoe extract used as an adjunct to conventional therapy for malignant disease, iscador helps in symptom control (e.g. pain, nausea and vomiting) thus improving quality of life. Treatment is available at the Royal London Homoeopathic Hospital (see also Chapter 9).

Other therapies
Hypnotherapy, autogenics and healing have also been used by cancer sufferers and their families to good effect. Seek expert advice.

Colds

What is it?

Colds are upper respiratory tract viral illnesses causing raised temperature, runny nose, sore throat, aches and pains, and cough. Antibiotics are ineffective against the causative viral agents. Colds probably occur more commonly in winter months because of central heating and a lack of ventilation. Children under 5 years old can expect to get 6–12 colds a year.

Cause

Many viruses are implicated, including adenovirus, respiratory syncitial virus (RSV) and rhinovirus.

Self-help

- Rest, fluids and paracetamol.
- Light diet, e.g. soups, bread.
- Stop smoking.
- 'TLC' (tender loving care).
- Most viral infections will last 7–10 days.

Conventional treatment

Reassurance and confirmation of the illness is all that is usually required.

Secondary bacterial infection is usually present if the symptoms go on for *more* than 7–10 days, the sputum is thick and discoloured all day, temperatures are constant, there is shortness of breath or if there is any extreme pain, e.g. in the throat and ears. These signs usually indicate bronchitis, tonsillitis or middle-ear infection and may need to be treated with antibiotics.

Complementary therapy

Acupuncture
Regular top-ups may help relieve shortness of breath and wheeze in chronic bronchitis.

Homoeopathy
Aconite, belladonna, nat. mur., merc. sol. or gelsemium, depending on symptoms (dose – 6C three times daily).

Herbal medicine
Excellent for relief of symptoms. Treat with chamomile or elder-flower tea, salt-water gargles, and honey, lemon and garlic in hot water as a cough mixture and gargle.

Aromatherapy
Oils for inhalation, massage or bathing: eucalyptus, sandalwood and hyssop.

Nutrition
Vitamin C 500 mg four times daily may shorten the length of a cold. Increase vitamin C levels through increased natural intake, especially orange, grapefruit and cranberry juice. Zinc lozenges may prevent colds but can have an unpleasant taste. Do not overdose.

Cystitis

What is it?

Cystitis is an inflammation of the lining of the bladder and urethra. It is most common in women, but children and men can suffer also. Symptoms include burning on urination (dysuria), passing water often (frequency), an urgent need to urinate (urgency), abdominal pain, and offensive and cloudy urine. High back pain, loin pain, chills, nausea and vomiting may indicate a kidney infection.

Causes

Cystitis is mainly due to ascending infection from the vagina through the urethra and into the bladder. Men are protected by the fact that they have a much longer urethra – physically it is more difficult for bacteria to infect the bladder.

The condition can occur several times a year for many women, often brought on by sexual intercourse, periods and intercurrent infection. Research suggests that these women may carry large numbers of abnormal organisms for long periods on their vulva, perhaps owing to a lack in local defence mechanisms. The most common organism causing cystitis is *Escherichia coli*, – a normal resident in the bowel.

Symptoms can also occur without bladder or urethral infection. Bruising through sexual intercourse, vaginal infections and sexually transmitted diseases (e.g. gonorrhoea, chlamydial infection) can cause identical symptoms.

Self-help

- Increase fluid intake so that the urine is clear.
- Urinate regularly – do not 'keep it in'.
- If urinating is very painful, try passing urine in a warm bath.
- Change the acidity of the urine by drinking a solution of bicarbonate of soda (a level teaspoon in a glass of water) three times daily. Over-the-counter powders are also available which have the same effect, e.g. Cymalon or potassium citrate mixture (avoid these if taking blood pressure medication).
- Avoid acidic fruits and drinks (e.g. orange juice).
- Paracetamol or ibuprofen regularly will settle the pain.
- A hot-water bottle wrapped in a towel on the lower abdomen will help ease abdominal discomfort.

Prevention

- Drink fluids regularly, keep the urine clear – especially on hot days.
- Urinate before *and* after sexual intercourse.
- Wipe from front to back after opening bowels.

- Wash the perineal area regularly, especially after opening bowels. However, *avoid* strong soaps, vaginal douches and vaginal deodorants.
- Avoid wearing tights and jeans. Stockings, loose trousers or skirts are better.
- Use a lubricant (e.g. KY jelly) if vaginal dryness may be a problem. This will also prevent urethral bruising.
- Reconsider using the diaphragm, or get a new one. Bacteria may colonize a diaphragm and infect the bladder after insertion.
- For chronic cystitis, use sanitary towels instead of tampons.

Conventional treatment

A general practitioner will test the urine for infection with a chemical stick (Dipstix). If the urine is cloudy or the Dipstix indicates protein, white cells, nitrite and blood, the GP will treat the infection with a 3–5 day course of antibiotics, e.g. trimethoprim, cephalexin or nitrofurantoin.

A midstream urine (MSU) sample may also be sent to the local hospital laboratory to identify the exact organism causing the infection. This is routine for a first infection or if the diagnosis of cystitis is doubtful.

First infections in children and men are always investigated further to eliminate any serious cause of disease.

Women who suffer from chronic cystitis may be given low-dose antibiotics to be taken for an indefinite period.

Complementary therapy

Acupressure
Press on points for 1–2 minutes:
Stomach 29 (2 fingerbreadths either side of the midline and 4 fingerbreadths below the navel).

Homoeopathy
Treat with one tablet hourly (10 doses maximum) as follows:
general symptoms: cantharis 30C, apis 30C, nux 6C
cystitis after intercourse: staphisagria 6C
abdomen burning, chilly: arsenicum 6C.

Herbal medicine
Yarrow tea, chamomile tea and barley water sipped regularly through the day will help ease symptoms.

Adding yarrow, calendula or marigold to a bath will ease back and abdominal symptoms (boil 100 g of herb in a 4 litres of water, drain and add to bath).

Naturopathy and nutrition
Practitioners will advise on self-help measures as above and on allergy testing, the role of *Candida*, juicing and supplements.

Cranberry juice contains vitamin C and quinolic acid which may help fight infection. Drink a glass four or five times daily.

High-dose vitamin C (1000 mg) taken daily will increase the acidity of the urine and stop bacterial growth. (Note: some antibiotics do not work in acidic urine – patients should inform their doctor if they are taking vitamin C supplements.)

Aromatherapy
Adding oils such as sandalwood to a warm bath will ease discomfort.

Eczema

What is it?

Eczema is a superficial inflammation of the skin with varying degrees of redness, blistering, oozing, crusting, scaling and itch; it is often known as dermatitis. Atopic eczema usually starts in childhood and is probably the most common type of eczema. Contact eczema or dermatitis is an allergic response to substances in contact with the skin. Eczema, asthma, allergic rhinitis and hay fever often occur together.

Cause

Childhood eczema (and asthma) has increased progressively since the 1980s. Factors implicated are increasing environmental pollution and processed foods. These may diminish the immune system and amplify any minor allergic or genetic predisposition.

Specific foods may also be implicated in children: these include dairy products, eggs, colourings, preservatives, lamb, chicken, soya, nuts and wheat. This sensitivity is probably mediated through a reaction in the gut wall. There is no strong evidence to implicate food sensitivities in adult eczema.

Symptoms often vary with weather (some forms of eczema improve in the sun), emotions, stress and intercurrent infection.

Self-help

- Exclusion diets – can take 6–8 weeks to show a sustained improvement. Such diets often work best in children under 2 years of age; seek expert help, e.g. from a dietician or nutritionist.
- Eczema can be aggravated by dry air – put a wet towel over radiators or leave a bowl of water in the room.
- Cotton clothing is better and more comfortable than polyester or wool for eczema sufferers.
- Avoid scratching, especially at night. Babies may need scratch mittens. Scratching damages skin, releasing chemicals that cause even more itching. For an irresistible itch, rubbing is better than scratching.
- Cold, wet dressings (with water or milk) can ease the heat and itch of an acute eczematous rash.
- Avoid soap. Wash instead with emollients such as aqueous cream, E45.
- Bathe in lukewarm water. Bathing reduces the chances of infection and helps keep the skin soft.
- Apply regular moisturizers (aqueous cream, E45, etc.) as often as possible, especially after bathing.
- For contact dermatitis – avoid nickel (jewellery is the most common source: nickel dermatitis is 10 times more common in women than in men), antiperspirants, solvents, polishes and anything else that may be implicated.
- For hand dermatitis: keep the hands warm and dry, and use cotton-lined gloves for peeling fruit and vegetables, washing up, handling other irritants, and shampooing hair.
- Over-the-counter medicines (e.g. 0.5% or 1% hydrocortisone, a mild steroid cream) applied twice daily may help reduce inflammation and itch. For babies, seek medical advice before treating with steroid creams. Calamine lotion helps cool itchy, oozing rashes.
- Join an eczema society:

  National Eczema Society
  Tavistock House East
  Tavistock Square
  London WC1H 9SR
  Tel. 0171 388 4097

Conventional treatment

Emollients, bath oils and steroid creams are the mainstays of therapy. Steroid creams are usually prescribed in increasing strengths.

They are a short-term measure only and can have potential adverse effects if used without proper medical guidance. Ideally steroids should be applied for 5 days followed by a 2-day rest ('never at weekends') and repeated until the acute eczema has resolved.

Antibiotics are used for infected eczema.

Antihistamines (e.g. chlorpheniramine, trimeprazine) help relieve itch and allow children to sleep at night.

Oil of evening primrose may help children with itch, scaling and overall severity.

Complementary therapy

Homoeopathy
Patients often report excellent results. For children's eczema, use pulsatilla 6C four times daily. For adults, use sulphur 6C four times daily.

Seek expert help.

Traditional Chinese herbalism
Some results have been so impressive that specialists at the Great Ormond Street Hospital have started to carry out research into this therapy. Patients often drink bitter tea made from herbal tea-bags.

Seek expert help only (see Chapter 4).

Hypnosis
Hypnosis may help adults and children with severe itching and sleep disturbance.

Acupuncture
Acupuncture may decrease the severity and frequency of acute attacks. Needling is unsuitable for young children.

Naturopathy and nutrition
Dietary advice and fasting may be advised.

Herbal medicine
Teas made from marigold, nettle and chamomile may help if taken regularly.

Aromatherapy
Sandalwood and fennel oils may help. Lotions made up from aromatic oils are occasionally applied directly to the eczematous area – seek expert help. Patients need to exercise caution as some oils will exacerbate eczema.

Hay fever

What is it?

Hay fever is an allergic reaction to pollen. It is most common in spring and summer, occurring occasionally in autumn. Symptoms include sneezing; red, sore, itchy, watery eyes; runny nose; itchy throat; headaches and wheezing.

Cause

    spring: tree pollen (e.g. oak, elm, alder, birch)
    summer: grass pollens
    autumn: ragweed pollens.

The disease can start at almost any age, but is most common in young adults. There is a hereditary pattern, especially if asthma, rhinitis or eczema runs in the family.

Self-help

- Keep indoors on high-pollen days.
- Wear a mouth and nose mask if going outside.
- Wearing petroleum jelly (Vaseline) around the nose helps trap pollen.
- Wear sunglasses. Use regular soothing eye-baths.

Conventional treatment

- Antihistamines in the form of of tablets (e.g. terfenadine, loratadine or cetirizine), anti-inflammatory nasal sprays (e.g. beclomethasone) and eye drops (e.g. sodium cromoglycate) are usually prescribed for the entire season.

Complementary therapies

Acupuncture
Acupuncture is useful as a preventive measure. Try to get in four to six treatments before the hay fever season starts.

Homoeopathy
For prevention, allium ceps and phosphorus 6C three times daily taken regularly through the season will help.

For acute symptoms, take dulcamara, gelsemium and arsenicum 6C every 2 hours up to 10 doses.

Enzyme-potentiated desensitization
See Chapter 9.

Aromatherapy
Use a few drops of hyssop or eucalyptus on a handkerchief and inhale.

Chinese herbal medicine
May give particularly good results in some individuals – seek expert advice.

Hypertension

What is it?

Hypertension is defined as elevation of systolic and/or diastolic blood pressure. This pressure is normally expressed as (for example) 120/80 mmHg. The upper is systolic, the lower is diastolic. Ideally systolic pressure should be less than 170 mmHg and diastolic less than 95 mmHg.

Control is essential to avoid long-term problems such as myocardial infarction (heart attack), strokes and kidney failure.

Typically, patients have no symptoms of hypertension.

Causes

In primary (or idiopathic) hypertension – the vast majority of cases – the cause is unknown. Secondary hypertension may be caused by kidney disease, metabolic problems, high alcohol intake and the oral contraceptive pill.

Self-help

Stop smoking, lose weight, reduce alcohol, salt and caffeine intake, commence or increase exercise, reduce stress.

Conventional treatment

The type of treatment depends on age and blood pressure. Blood pressure is monitored regularly, and medication (such as diuretics, beta-blockers, calcium antagonists or angiotensin-converting enzyme (ACE) inhibitors is prescribed accordingly.

Complementary therapy

It is vital to continue with conventional treatment while trying complementary therapy. If blood pressure does come down, only reduce medication under strict medical supervision.

Most therapies are good for relaxation and relief of stress only. Especially recommended are acupuncture, massage, reflexology and autogenics.

Naturopaths, homoeopaths, herbalists and ayurvedic practitioners will often give self-help treatment as above.

Insomnia

What is it?

Difficulty in sleeping or a disturbance in the sleep pattern may take various forms, including delay in getting to sleep, waking on several occasions, long periods without sleep (lying awake all night) and waking too early.

Causes

The cause may be physiological – some people need little sleep, others much more. An elderly person often needs less sleep than someone younger and more active. Other causes include:

overeating, especially consumption of stimulants such as alcohol and caffeine
psychological problems: anxiety, bereavement, marital difficulties, work problems, depression, etc.
change in environment – travel, noise, odd surroundings
jet-lag.

Self-help

- Go to bed when tired, avoid cat-napping through the day.
- Make time for some gentle exercise in the afternoon or early evening, but not just before going to bed.
- Sleep in a dark, quiet, well-ventilated room on a comfortable bed.
- It is better to get up and do something than lie in bed tossing and turning.
- Take up a regular bedtime routine, e.g. playing soft music, reading, taking a warm bath.
- A small milky drink will help, but avoid stimulants such as alcohol, tea, coffee and cola.
- Avoid drinking too much fluid before bedtime if bladder capacity is poor.
- Wake up at the same time each morning.
- Learn and practise relaxation techniques.

Conventional treatment

Most general practitioners will give general advice similar to above. Doctors are very reluctant to start patients on sleeping tablets because of their addictive potential and side-effects (drowsiness during the day, agitation, and difficulty in carrying out routine daytime tasks). *If* tablets are prescribed it is usually for 7–10 days to help the patient re-establish a normal sleep pattern.

Patients with underlying depression or anxiety often do better on sedative antidepresssants taken at night, e.g. amitriptyline 10–25 mg.

Complementary therapy

Acupressure
Press on points for 1–2 minutes:
   Spleen 6
   Colon 4
For point location, see Chapter 2.

Acupuncture
Four to six weekly treatments may help to re-establish a disturbed sleep pattern.

Homoeopathy
Aconite 30C, arnica 30C, chamomile 30C or rhus 30C, given
30 minutes to 1 hour before bedtime.

Herbal medicine
Tea or infusions made from lavender, rosemary, passiflora or
chamomile taken before bedtime will help relaxation and reduce
anxiety.

Aromatherapy and massage
A gentle massage with jasmine, sandalwood, chamomile or lavender
will calm tense muscles and aid relaxation. The oils can also be used
in a bath.

Reflexology
A general massage of the feet will help relaxation and reduce
anxiety.

Meditation
Visualization and imagery especially work well in insomnia.
Regular meditation is an excellent relaxation technique that is
easy to learn.

Other therapies
Hypnotherapy, autogenics and biofeedback can all be helpful.

Irritable bowel syndrome

What is it?

Irritable bowel syndrome (IBS) is a disruption of the smooth co-
ordination of the contractions of the bowel muscle, causing spasmodic abdominal pains (colic), alternating diarrhoea and constipation, pellet stools and bloating. The female to male ratio is 3 : 1.
    This syndrome is the probable cause of half of all abdominal
complaints. It usually resolves spontaneously by early middle age.

Cause

Psychological factors, diet, hormones or drugs may aggravate an
inherited gastrointestinal tendency. Stress and depression have a
particularly severe effect on IBS.

Self-help

- A stress and food diary may help connect symptoms with food sensitivities and specific stresses.
- Learning relaxation and meditation techniques with the help of tapes or books and classes, and better stress management, may have a significant effect on symptoms.
- Increase the amount of fibre in the diet by eating bran, vegetables and fruit.
- Increase fluid intake: drink 6–8 average-sized glassfuls daily.
- Chew food properly, eat slowly. Frequent meals are easier to digest and pose less strain on the gastrointestinal system than two or three large meals a day.
- Avoid stimulants such as coffee, alcohol, cola and tobacco.
- Fat can worsen IBS – decrease intake of fried or oily foods.
- Dairy products and wheat can worsen symptoms. Try cutting these out gradually or try gluten-free products. Some patients may not have IBS but may simply be lactose intolerant; milk would worsen symptoms.
- Avoid foods that cause 'gas', e.g. beans, pulses, cabbage, onions, brussel sprouts and broccoli.
- Increase intake of chicken and fish, avoid red meat.
- Avoid tomatoes and other seed-containing foods.
- Exercise often helps to cut down the frequency and severity of attacks.
- For acute symptoms, simple analgesics such as paracetamol and ibuprofen may help.
- Join the IBS Network; this organization publishes *Gut Reaction*, a newsletter by and, for sufferers of IBS:

> IBS Network
> St John's House
> Hither Green Hospital
> Hither Green Lane
> London SE13 6RU
> Tel. 0181 698 4611 (ext. 8194)

Conventional treatment

Dietary advice (as above) given in leaflets available from doctors form the mainstay of treatment.

Supplementation of dietary fibre with bulking agents such as Fybogel. For severe symptoms (e.g. colic), antispasmodics such as mebeverine or hyoscine butylbromide will relax the smooth muscle in the intestinal wall and ease pain and bloating.

Thorough investigation of symptoms is essential if disease begins in middle age or later, to exclude serious bowel problems.

Complementary therapy

Acupressure
Press on points for 1–2 minutes:
  Colon 4
  Liver 3
For point location, see Chapter 2.

Acupuncture
Helps to reduce stress and calm an overactive bowel.

Homoeopathy
Colocynth 6C, argent. nit. 6C, four times daily.

Herbal Medicine
Teas made from peppermint, fennel or cardamom should be sipped slowly throughout the day.

Naturopathy and nutrition
Self-help advice as above. Vitamin supplements such as thiamine and vitamin C may also be prescribed.

Meditation
Visualization techniques work especially well.

Other therapies
Hypnosis, aromatherapy and biofeedback may help. Chinese herbal medicine can be particularly effective – seek expert advice.

Labour pain

What is it?

Labour is a progressive process that leads to the successful delivery of the baby and placenta. There are three main stages:

- First stage: regular painful contractions, increasing in intensity. The cervix opens up and stretches to create a smooth birth canal with the vagina (effacement). This stage lasts between 6 hours and 24 hours.

- Second stage: once the cervix is fully dilated, the mother will have the urge to push with contractions. The baby is usually delivered within 15–60 minutes.
- Third stage: The afterbirth or placenta is delivered within 5–10 minutes.

Cause

Labour pain is caused by cervical stretching. Contraction of the womb causes pain fibres to be squeezed, and stretches the muscle, ligaments and tendons of the pelvis and the nerve fibres intimate with them. There is a reduction in the arterial blood flow of muscle fibres in the womb on contraction.

Stretching and pressure on the tissues and nerve fibres of the lower pelvis and vagina occur as the baby descends. The pain is worse if the baby is disproportionately large or the woman has a small pelvis.

Other factors affecting pain levels in labour are the number of previous births, anxiety, presence of a partner, age (less pain in younger mothers), social and family background (e.g. mother's childbirth experiences), culture, periods (women with less period pain may have less labour pains), ability to relax and how much the mother understands pregnancy and labour.

Self-help

- Regular pelvic floor exercises throughout pregnancy may help reduce labour pain and perineal tearing.
- Oiling the perineal area in the month before labour may help prevent tearing.
- Learn correct breathing and relaxation techniques taught in antenatal classes by midwives, the National Childbirth Trust (NCT) and the Active Birth Movement. Regularly practising these techniques will make them second nature during labour itself.
- Find out all about pregnancy and labour. Understand the processes and learn what to expect. Contact the NCT or the Active Birth Centre for classes:

  Active Birth Centre
  Bickerton House
  Bickerton Road
  London N19 5JT
  Tel. 0171 561 9006

National Childbirth Trust
Alexandra House
Oldham Terrace
London W3 6NH
Tel. 0181 992 8637

Conventional treatment

Transcutaneous electrical nerve stimulation (TENS) is now so common that it should be classed as a conventional treatment. Four electrodes are placed on the middle and lower back with the machine carried in a pouch on the side. The patient can turn the current up or down according to the level of pain she is experiencing. The mechanism of action of TENS is similar to acupuncture. It can be used for labour pain as well as for backache in late pregnancy. Community midwives and hospitals may be able to provide TENS units; alternatively the units can be hired (£25–30 per month).

Other methods of pain relief include nitrous oxide and oxygen (Entonox) or 'gas and air'. This works within two or three breaths, and is almost universally used.

Pcthidine injections work within 15–30 minutes and are very popular, but can affect the baby if given late in labour. Meptazinol (Meptid) injection is similar to pethidine, but is seldom used in the UK.

Epidural anaesthesia is used by almost one-third of women. It provides the best pain relief of conventional methods but can increase the likelihood of an assisted delivery (e.g. forceps, vacuum).

Pudendal block, an injection of lignocaine around the pudendal nerve to numb the tissues of the perineum, is often used in assisted deliveries (forceps or vacuum) or before an episiotomy is made.

Complementary therapy

Acupressure
Press on points for 1–2 miutes at a time:
   Colon 4
   Liver 3
   Spleen 6
For point location see Chapter 2.

Acupuncture
Acupuncture may be used in the first stage of labour. Electro-acupuncture is particularly helpful. It can be costly because of the

time involved; however, some midwives may learn these techniques in the near future.

Homoeopathy

- Belladonna 30C, coffea 30C, kali. carb. 30C every 5–10 minutes, 10 doses maximum.
- Arnica 30C for post-delivery bruising, every 2–3 hours.
- Arnica solution (10 drops in 250 ml of water) – bathe bruised areas three or four times daily.

Homoeopathic treatment is safe for mother and child throughout pregnancy and during the post-natal period.

Hypnotherapy
Hypnotherapy works well for pain control and relaxation. Self-hypnosis needs to be practised regularly if it is to be used successfully in labour.

Aromatherapy
Aromatherapy has been used successfully in some maternity units. Massage in oils 10–15 minutes hourly to relax muscles, ease pain and help anxiety. Bathing with a few drops of aromatic oils will also help relaxation and ease tension in muscles.

See Chapter 7 for recommended oils in pregnancy and labour.

Massage
Massage helps relax muscles and eases anxiety. Massage of the shoulders, neck, lower back and buttocks by a partner is particularly helpful.

Hydrotherapy
Many companies hire out 'birthing pools' and some hospitals have them on site. Pools are also available to hire from the Active Birth Centre (address above). However, a large bath will suffice.

The woman feels lighter, more mobile and relaxed. There is less pressure on the abdomen which eases pain and reduces anxiety. Most women get out of the pool when actually delivering their babies.

Reflexology
Reflexology is given by an increasing number of midwives but can easily be administered by a partner. It helps relaxation and eases pain.

Bach flower remedies
A few drops of Rescue Remedy on the tongue may help anxiety and
pain.

Meditation
Visualization and imagery may help relaxation and reduce pain. It
is advisable to practise these techniques throughout pregnancy.

Autogenics
With regular practice, autogenics may help with pain relief and
relaxation in pregnancy, labour and after delivery. See Chapter 6
for examples of exercises.

Menopausal problems

What is it?

The cessation of menstruation (for 1 year) as a result of decreasing
ovarian function usually occurs between the ages of 48 and 52
years, but some women can be as young as 35. Symptoms are hot
flushes, sweating, fatigue, irritability, insomnia, anxiety, palpitations, nausea, constipation, diarrhoea, joint pains, muscular
aches, painful intercourse, urinary incontinence and cystitis.

Women who have had surgical removal or radiotherapy of their
ovaries will also experience similar symptoms.

Cause

Decreasing ovarian function reduces oestrogen production. This in
turn causes levels of pituitary gonadotrophins – follicle stimulating
hormone (FSH), and luteinizing hormone (LH) – to rise substantially. These biochemical changes cause the typical menopausal
symptoms. Psychological and social factors, such as ageing, loss of
central family role and grown-up children, also play a part in symp-
tomology.

Premenopausally women are protected against osteoporosis and
ischaemic heart disease by circulating oestrogens. After the menopause the incidence of heart disease in women increases rapidly to
match that of men.

Self-help

- Avoid symptom triggers that may bring on hot flushes, e.g. emotional upset, hot, spicy food and warm rooms.

- Learn simple relaxation techniques to avoid emotional upsets.
- Eat small meals and drink plenty of fluids to help the body regulate temperature more easily.
- Decrease alcohol and caffeine intake.
- To help slow down osteoporosis, stop smoking, increase calcium supplements and exercise regularly.
- Continue with regular sexual intercourse (at least once weekly). Sexual activity may stimulate failing ovaries and help increase oestrogen levels.
- For vaginal dryness, use a good lubricant such as KY jelly. This also cuts down the likelihood of post-coital cystitis.
- Pelvic floor exercises will help prevent urinary incontinence and increase the tone of vaginal muscles.

Conventional treatment

The aim of treatment is to relieve symptoms and prevent osteoporosis, heart disease and strokes. Hormone replacement therapy (HRT) is very effective in controlling menopausal symptoms, particularly flushing, sweating and insomnia. The hormones can be given as tablets, patches, gels or intra-abdominal implants. Regular periods will recommence with HRT in women who have not had a hysterectomy. For this reason many women give up HRT within a few months of starting.

Osteoporosis is a major problem after the menopause: 1–3% of a woman's bone mass is lost per year, and by the age of 70 years a women will have lost 50% of her bone mass. Untreated, these women will have an increased risk of fractures (especially of the hip, wrist and vertebral bones).

Osteoporosis is more likely if the woman has a family history of the condition, smokes, drinks alcohol and caffeine to excess, takes little exercise, has low body weight and poor nutrition, is of European or Asian origin, is on long-term steroid therapy or has had an early menopause. For osteoporosis prevention, HRT should be given for a minimum of 5 years, ideally for 10 years in those with normal onset menopause. For early menopause, i.e. late 30s or early 40s, treatment needs to be until age 60 years.

Vaginal dryness may be treated by direct application of oestrogen gels.

In addition to prescribing HRT the doctor will also check blood pressure and arrange for a mammogram (if the woman is over 50), a vaginal examination (to exclude uterine and ovarian masses) and a cervical smear.

Complementary therapy

Acupressure
Press on points for 1–2 minutes:
   Yintang
   Kidney 6 (1 fingerbreadth below the inner ankle bone)
For point location see Chapter 2.

Acupuncture
Acupuncture is helpful for anxiety, palpitations, insomnia and aching joints and muscles.

Homoeopathy
Dose twice daily as follows:
   hot flushes: kali. carb. 30C, graphites 30C, lachesis 30C
   irritability: pulsatilla 30C
   sweating: sepia 30C.

Herbal medicine
Tea or infusions made from chamomile, raspberry leaf, agnus castus and motherwort, sipped regularly throughout the day will help symptoms.

Aromatherapy and massage
Sage, cypress, chamomile and marigold oils used in a massage, bath or as an inhalation will reduce anxiety and help night sweats.

Naturopathy and nutrition
Self-help measures as above will be advised. Supplementation may also be recommended:
   vitamin C 1000 mg daily
   vitamin E 40–50 mg daily
   calcium 1000 mg daily for women on HRT, 1500 mg for untreated women
   vitamin D 600 units twice daily.

Other therapies
Reflexology, Bach flower remedies, autogenics and hypnotherapy will aid anxiety, insomnia and hot flushes.

Migraine and headache

What is it?

The vast majority of headaches are muscle contraction (or tension) headaches, cluster headaches, migraine or head pain of unknown origin. Muscle tension headaches are usually intermittent, bi-frontal or general, and patients describe a feeling of a tight band around the head. These headaches tend to worsen towards the end of the day and are more common in individuals susceptible to stress.

Migraines are throbbing in nature and begin around the eyes and spread to involve one or both sides of the head. There is often photophobia (dislike of bright light), nausea and vomiting. Similar periodic attacks occur over time (days or months). In the few hours or days before a migraine occurs, sufferers may feel very tired or very full of energy. Some crave food – sweets in particular. One in 10 migraine sufferers has a warning 'aura' which occurs before the headache starts. This may include flashing lights or zigzag lines which move across the eyes, as well as blank spots (scotomas) on looking at objects. Some may experience numbness or loss of function of one side of their body during an attack (hemiparesis).

Migraine usually begins between the ages of 10 years and 30 years. Women suffer more than men. There is a family history of the condition in over 50% of cases.

Cluster headaches are paroxysmal attacks that may occur every day for weeks or months, in 'clusters'. The pain is severe, typically around or behind one eye, temple and face; 90% of sufferers are men.

Cause

Muscle contraction headaches are caused by 'strain' of the muscles around the head, neck and shoulders due to either physical or emotional stresses.

Migraine may be due to a disturbance in cranial blood flow. The 'aura' (lights and visual disturbances) of migraine is probably due to constriction of blood vessels. This is followed by a throbbing headache as vessels dilate and blood pours into the brain.

Cluster headaches may be due to hormonal or genetic factors. Studies are being carried out on a possible link with testosterone. There may be a link with nicotine – the majority of male sufferers are heavy smokers.

Self-help

- Take painkillers at the *first sign* of a headache.
- Have a nap in a dark, quiet room.
- A tight headband will decrease scalp blood flow and lessen throbbing headaches.

Prevention

Changes in eating habits or certain activities may trigger migraine attacks – monitor for possible trigger factors:

- Diet: chocolate, cheese, fried food, red wine, dieting.
- Emotions: tension, anger, depression.
- Change of routine: excitement, holiday and travel, shift work, change of job, oversleeping.
- Hormone changes: periods, the menopause, the pill.
- Others: bright sunlight, flickering lights, noise, strong smells.

Facial calisthenic exercises will help relax the muscles and prevent tension headaches (e.g. raise eyebrows together, raise eyebrows separately, make faces, yawn). Sleeping on the side or back puts less strain on neck muscles. Avoid chewing gum – the repetitive action can cause muscle tension.

Join a migraine association:

British Migraine Association
178A High Road
Byfleet
West Byfleet
Surrey KT14 7ED
Tel. 01932 352468

Conventional treatment

A full history and examination including blood pressure and fundoscopy (visualization of the retina) is important to exclude serious causes and reassure the patient.

Simple analgesia, e.g. co-proxamol, may be sufficient. For acute migraines use analgesic formulations containing antiemetics, e.g. Migraleve, Migravess and Paramax. Alternatively sumatriptan may 'switch off' a migrainous attack – given by tablet or subcutaneous injection (no more than two injections or three 100-mg tablets in 24 hours).

For migraine prevention, beta-blockers, pizotifen and low-dose antidepressants may help.

Low-dose antidepressants (e.g. 10–25 mg of amitriptyline) often work very well in tension headaches.

Complementary therapy

Acupressure
Press on points for 1–2 minutes:
   Colon 4
   Liver 2
For point location see Chapter 2.

Acupuncture
Acupuncture is excellent for migraine; it cuts down the frequency and severity of attacks. Regular top-ups (every 1–6 months) are advisable. However, it does not seem to work well for cluster headaches.

Homoeopathy
Treat as follows:
   migraine: nat. mur. 6C, pulsatilla 6C
   tension headaches: arnica 30C, ignatia 6C.
Give one dose every 15 minutes during an attack, up to 10 doses. Seek expert help for severe, complex migraines.

Herbal medicine
For migraine prevention:
   tea made from feverfew or chamomile sipped regularly
   feverfew 200mg daily in tablet form.
Benefits are not usually seen before 6 weeks.

Aromatherapy and massage
These therapies are a good combination for releasing muscle tensions and general relaxation.

Osteopathy and chiropractice
Certain manipulative techniques can help tension headaches.

Reflexology
The reflexes corresponding to all of the head are found in the big toes. Squeezing the tip of the big toe may relieve a migrainous attack.

Naturopathy and nutrition
Avoid trigger factors and follow the self-help advice given above. Massage, fasting and body cleansing may all be recommended to help prevent headaches.

Self-hypnosis
Self-hypnosis works well for tension headaches and can decrease frequency of migraine attacks.

Biofeedback
Biofeedback is useful for all types of headaches.

Meditation
Visualization and imagery may help tension headaches.

Post-viral fatigue syndrome

What is it?

Post-viral fatigue (PVF) syndrome is also known as chronic fatigue syndrome (CFS) or myalgic encephalomyelitis (ME). It is a chronic condition characterized by some or all of the following symptoms: persistent or relapsing fatigue, depression, poor concentration, poor short-term memory, muscular aches, joint pains, headaches, enlarged lymph glands, sleep disturbance, tinnitus, laryngitis and irritable bowel syndrome.

The condition starts within a few days or weeks of a typical flu-like viral illness or glandular fever. Exacerbations occur following overexertion or intercurrent infection. The syndrome usually lasts over 6 months with spontaneous recovery. Some patients are affected for several years, sometimes for life, with severe debility (about 5%).

Between 150 000 and 200 000 people are affected in the UK, and up to half a million in America. The syndrome is rare below the age of 10 years or above 50 years; occurring mainly in adults and adolescents.

Most investigations are normal and sufferers are often labelled as neurotic. Little progress has been made in definitive treatment, although research has shown the presence of antiviral antibodies, low red cell magnesium levels and muscle abnormalities in some sufferers.

Cause

The syndrome is probably multifactorial; no single cause has been identified. Possible factors involved include:

- Viral infection – the Epstein–Barr virus, which causes glandular fever, may be involved. Other viral triggers include those causing hepatitis and meningitis.
- Personality – patients are often 'type A', i.e. competitive and perfectionist.
- Psychological problems – 50–65% of patients have a co-existing psychiatric disorder, e.g. depression, anxiety.
- High levels of stress.
- Significant life events – e.g. bereavement, job loss, major operation or illness.
- Abnormalities of endocrine secretion – cortisol levels in PVF syndrome tend to be low.

Self-help

- Seek an accurate diagnosis. Not all complex and confusing symptom patterns are PVF syndrome.
- Decrease stress, increase periods of relaxation. Rest should be taken according to a daily timetable and *not* according to symptoms.
- A graded exercise programme may help some sufferers:
    choose targets, not distances, e.g. 'walk to the shops' or 'sit in the garden three times a day', *not* 'walk 250 metres' or 'cycle for 20 minutes'.
    choose targets consistent with *current* levels of fitness and activity.
- Stop smoking and reduce alcohol intake.
- Counselling may help patients to come to terms with the illness.
- Join a society or self-help group:

    ME Action Campaign
    PO Box 1302
    Wells
    Somerset BA5 2WE
    Tel. 01749 670577

ME Association
Stanhope House
High Street
Stanford-le-Hope
Essex SS17 0HA
Tel. 01375 642466

Conventional treatment

Basic investigations are required to rule out other serious disease. Reassurance, advice and counselling are the basis of treatment, with occasional use of sleeping tablets and painkillers.

Cognitive behavioural therapy aims to reduce erratic activity patterns and avoidance behaviour. Eventually a graded exercise programme can be introduced with the psychologist and doctor working with the patient.

Small doses of antidepressants (e.g. amitriptyline 10–25 mg) at night often help. The use of selective serotonin re-uptake inhibitors (SSRIs) such as fluoxetine and paroxetine may help patients with a significant depressive element.

Patients are encouraged to understand the illness, and to think of treatment in terms of rehabilitation and management of symptoms. Aiming at a 'cure' may lead to frustration, depression and anxiety and may be counterproductive. However, most patients *do* get better.

Complementary therapy

Acupuncture
Regular sessions may boost the immune system and help in relaxation.

Acupressure
Press on each point for 1–2 minutes:
   Spleen 6
   Colon 4.
For point location see Chapter 2.

Homoeopathy
China 30C twice daily for 3 days may help. Seek expert help for specific remedies.

Herbal medicine
Teas or infusions of calendula, marigold, chamomile and rosemary may help symptoms.

Aromatherapy
Regular massage with basil, sage, lavender or jasmine will help muscular aches.

Hydrotherapy
Daily cold baths or showers may boost the immune system and help symptoms.

Magnesium injections
In patients with low red cell magnesium levels, intramuscular magnesium injections have helped muscle aches and fatigue.

Naturopathy and nutrition
The patient is advised about healthy eating and self-help. Vitamins and mineral supplements may help boost the immune system, especially vitamin B complex, magnesium and zinc.

Some practitioners may undertake treatment of generalized candidiasis, especially in the gastrointestinal system, by regular medication; this remains a controversial issue with the medical profession.

Oil of evening primrose has helped up to 70% of sufferers in clinical trials.

Other therapies
Meditation, self-hypnosis, probiotics, reflexology, Bach flower remedies, ayureveda, Chinese herbal medicine and autogenics may all help.

Premenstrual tension and period pains

What is it?

Premenstrual tension (PMT) is an exaggerated response to the change in hormone levels during the monthly cycle. The condition can only be diagnosed if the woman has a few days of being completely symptom-free during the month – usually when bleeding starts.

Symptoms of PMT are weight gain, bloating, irritability, moodiness, anxiety, depression, tender breasts, headaches, backache, loss of libido and odd behavioural patterns.

The vast majority of women suffer from period pain (dysmenorrhoea). Typically, spasmodic abdominal pain is accompanied by backache for the first few days of a period. Occasionally the pain will last throughout the period.

Causes

Premenstrual tension is caused by a reaction to fluctuations of progesterone and oestrogen hormones during the menstrual cycle. If the hormones are in balance the woman may not suffer from PMT at all. If oestrogen levels predominate she may feel anxious, irritable and suffer bloating, fluid retention and weight gain. If progesterone is more dominant she may become depressed and fatigued.

Period pains are thought to occur as a result of uterine contractions and a relative decrease in the blood supply of the uterine muscles. These effects are probably mediated by prostaglandins produced in the lining of the uterus.

Self-help

- Avoid sugar, alcohol, caffeine and salt.
- Increase consumption of fresh fruit and vegetables.
- Decrease intake of dairy products – lactose can block the body's absorption of magnesium which helps regulate oestrogen levels.
- Reduce stress by learning simple relaxation techniques.
- Exercise – decreases fluid retention, releases endorphins that have a mood-enhancing effect. Ideally increase exercise 1–2 weeks before the onset of PMT.
- Increasing sleep may help with tiredness and irritability.

Conventional treatment

Treatment of PMT includes diuretics for fluid retention (for 2–5 days only of the cycle); hormonal manipulation (e.g. oral contraceptive pills, progesterone pills, vaginal pessaries) to eliminate cyclical changes; antidepressants in severely depressed or suicidal patients; and vitamin B_6 (pyridoxine) tablets.

Period pain is treated with simple analgesics such as co-proxamol and paracetamol/codeine drugs. Non-steroidal anti-inflammatory drugs such as mefanamic acid have antiprostaglandin effects and help pain relief; they work better if started 1–2 days before the onset of bleeding. Suppression of ovulation with the oral contraceptive pill is an alternative approach.

Complementary therapy

Acupressure
Press on points for 1–2 minutes:
period pain: Conception Vessel 4 (3 fingerbreadths below the umbilicus), Spleen 6
PMT: Colon 4, Liver 3, Spleen 6.
For point location see Chapter 2.

Acupuncture
Acupuncture is very good for period pain; it is best given 1 week before menstruation commences. It has had only limited success with PMT.

Homoeopathy
- Period pain:
    general period pain: belladonna 30C, chamomilla 30C
    spasmodic pain: mag. phos. 30C, cimicifuga 30C
    fluid retention: pulsatilla 30C
    Doses 4-hourly.
- Premenstrual tension:
    general PMT: nux 30C, sepia 30C
    irritable, oversensitive: causticum 30C
    depressed: lycopodium 30C
    fluid retention, tender breasts: nat. mur. 30C
    Dose two or three times daily, starting 1 day before symptoms are expected.

Herbal medicine
- Period pain: infusions or teas from wild yam, carraway and ginger root.
- PMT: agnus castus, chamomile tea.

Aromatherapy and massage
- Period pain: cypress, melissa, marjoram and aniseed.
- PMT: chamomile, melissa, sage, cypress and lavender.

Massage will ease tight muscles and tensions and may also help fluid retention. A warm bath with the oils will help relaxation.

Naturopathy and nutrition
Practitioners will give advice on diets and supplementation:

vitamin B_6 (pyridoxine) 50–100 mg daily for PMT symptoms
vitamin C 500 mg daily may relieve stress during PMT
vitamin E 40–50 mg daily relieves breast symptoms, anxiety and depression
vitamins A and D may help suppress PMT acne or oily skin
zinc 5 mg daily for general PMT symptoms
magnesium 1 tablet daily controls food cravings and stabilises moods
oil of evening primrose 1000 mg twice daily 2 days before the symptoms commence for general PMT symptoms.

Other therapies
Reflexology, Bach flower remedies, autogenics and hypnotherapy will also help.

Sinusitis

What is it?

The sinus cavities around the nose and eyes become blocked and infected. The symptoms may be all or some of the following: facial pain on stooping, facial congestion, runny or stuffy nose, raised temperature, watery eyes, sensation of a 'bad smell', discoloured nasal discharge.

Cause

Allergies to pollen, moulds, dust, animal dander, house dust mites and foodstuffs (e.g. egg, artificial colourants, wheat, milk, nuts, seafood) may all cause sinusitis, as may air pollution and stuffy office buildings ('sick building' syndrome).

Self-help

- Avoid culprit allergens and foods.
- Inhalations in a hot shower or over a bowl full of hot water.
- Drink extra fluids (this thins out the mucus).
- Humidify the home.
- Bathe nostrils with saline – sniff and blow one nostril at a time.
- Rubbing over the sinuses increases blood circulation and soothes.

- Apply moist heat over the sinuses, e.g. a warm, wet towel for 5 minutes.

Conventional treatment

Decongestant nasal sprays (maximum of 2 weeks) and/or antihistamine tablets or sprays will help to damp down the allergic process. Acute infections are treated with antibiotics.

Persistent sinusitis may require surgery to unblock and drain the sinuses. However, the recurrence rate tends to be high.

Complementary therapy

Acupuncture
Treatment involves needling points in the face. It is useful for facial pain, congestion and reducing mucus production.

Acupressure
Press on each point for 1–2 minutes:
Yintang (between the eyebrows)
Stomach 3 (one and a half fingerbreadths below the lower eyelid, on the cheekbone).

Homoeopathy
Homoeopathy is very useful. Give nat. mur., kali. bichrom., hepar. sulph. or pulsatilla depending on symptoms; dose 6C, one tablet six times daily.

Herbal medicine
Tea or infusion made from marsh-mallow.

Aromatherapy
Oils for use as inhalations: eucalyptus, pine.
Oils for use as massage: geranium, lavender.

Nutrition
Garlic, horseradish and cajun spice contain chemicals to thin and clear the mucus.

Chinese herbal medicine
May work particularly well in some patients – seek expert help.

Sports injury

What is it?

The term 'sports injury' covers strains, sprains, 'pulled' muscles and ligaments, shin splints and stress fractures ('sprain' is damage to ligaments; 'strain' is damage to muscles and tendons). Symptoms include pain, swelling, bruising and difficulty in weight-bearing. Most are soft-tissue injuries. In severe cases where there is an *inability* to weight-bear or bony tenderness, medical advice should be sought to exclude a fracture.

Cause

These injuries are most common in individuals who have just re-started exercise after a long break or those who have not adequately warmed up. Sudden overstretching of 'cold' soft tissues results in injury. Overuse or direct trauma can cause similar symptoms and signs.

Self-help

- For immediate action, remember the acronym 'RICE':
    R – **rest**: stop the activity
    I – apply **ice** regularly: for 15 minutes every 3–4 hours
    C – **compression**: apply a firm bandage or Tubigrip
    E – **elevate** the limb.
- Simple analgesia, for example with paracetamol, will help.
- Gentle exercise to stretch and relax muscles.
- When a bony injury has been excluded, follow the old casualty adage 'if it hurts, move it'.

Conventional treatment

Follow the 'RICE' procedure only if no bony injury is present. Give stronger analgesics if required.

Fractures and major ligament ruptures (causing an unstable joint) are treated at accident and emergency departments with advice to avoid weight-bearing, immobilization in plaster, and splinting. Major bony fractures may require surgery for internal fixation.

Physiotherapy may include stretching exercises and ultrasound therapy.

Complementary therapy

Acupressure
Acupressure is often too painful to perform. However, pressure for 1–2 minutes on Bladder 60 may help ankle and leg pain; Gallbladder 34 is used for knee pain.

For point location see Chapter 2.

Acupuncture
Acupuncture provides good relief for pain but little help for swelling and bruising. It complements well with physiotherapy.

Aromatherapy and massage
These therapies are useful for stretching and relaxing strained muscles. Avoid deep massage. Oils used are marjoram and sage.

Homoeopathy
For pain, bruising:
 arnica or hypericum cream
 arnica 30C tablets half-hourly, 10 doses maximum.

Thrush (candidiasis)

What is it?

Thrush is a fungal yeast infection; the most common area of infection is the vagina. *Candida* occurs naturally on the surface of the skin.

Cause

Infection only becomes a problem at times of lowered immunity or when conditions encourage the overgrowth of *Candida*. Typically the affected area of the body is sweaty, warm and poorly ventilated, e.g. vagina, mouth, groin and nappy area.

Self-help

- Wear stockings, skirts or loose cotton trousers. Avoid tights or tight clothing, especially in a warm climate.
- Avoid detergents, perfumed soaps, disinfectants in the bath.
- Wash the vulval area gently with a solution of 30 ml (2 tablespoons) of vinegar in 5 litres of water.

- Avoid antibiotics if possible. If necessary ask the doctor for medication to *prevent* thrush.

Conventional treatment

Treatment consists of measures as above, plus antifungal pessaries to be inserted into the vagina, and creams. Antifungal oral tablets are also available which have the advantge of being less messy. Partners are also treated and patients are advised to avoid sexual intercourse during therapy.

Complementary therapy

Many complementary practitioners such as naturopaths believe that generalized candidiasis is the cause of a great many ailments and may treat patients with high-dose antifungal tablets for months. This remains a highly contentious issue amongst orthodox doctors.

Aromatherapy
Tea tree oil on a tampon is an effective antifungal treatment.

Herbal medicine
A salt wash can be prepared by adding a tablespoon (15 ml) of salt to half a litre of water. Use this as a vaginal wash two or three times daily.

Homoeopathy
Oral thrush can be treated with capsicum 6C four times daily for 5 days. Treatment of vaginal thrush depends on symptoms: seek expert help.

Naturopathy and nutrition
Avoid yeast-containing foods (mushrooms, cheese).
Avoid sugar, starch and alcohol.
Avoid food or drinks containing colouring, flavouring or preservatives.
Avoid stimulants which trigger sugar release in the body, e.g. tea, coffee, cola and smoking.
Supplements of vitamins (e.g. B complex), minerals (zinc, selenium) and amino acids may strengthen the immune system.

Probiotics
Insert live natural yoghurt into the vagina twice daily. Increase the intake of lactobacilli by eating more live yoghurt. High-potency *Lactobacillus acidophilus* powder plus bifidobacteria powder can be taken as a dose of half to one teaspoonful of each in water three times daily.

11

Addictions

Complementary therapies for addiction

What is addiction?

Addiction is a style of living characterized by continuing use of and overwhelming physical and psychological involvement with a particular substance. Most 'addicts' seen in general practice are involved with hard drugs (heroin, cocaine, crack, LSD, amphetamines, barbiturates and Ecstasy), tranquillizers (e.g. sleeping tablets), cannabis, solvents, glue, alcohol and smoking. Addictions not usually seen as serious but which still obey the definition above include addiction to caffeine and foodstuffs such as chocolate.

The male to female ratio for alcoholism is 4 : 1. However; women appear to be catching up; 5–10% of drinkers may be dependent on alcohol.

One-third of adults in the UK are smokers; 90% believe it is bad for their health and 70% want to stop.

Cause

Addiction may be the result of personality traits, for instance the 'addictive' personality who gives in to frustration quickly, or the 'schizoid' personality who is isolated, shy and lonely.

Stress from work (or lack of it), marriage, illness, depression, etc. may be a cause, as may social and peer pressure, especially amongst teenagers.

Increasing ease of access to addictive substances is also a factor.

Self-help for alcohol addiction

- You need to acknowledge the problem. Use the 'CAGE' questionnaire:

C – have you ever thought you ought to **cut** down your drinking?

A – has anyone ever **annoyed** you by criticizing your drinking?

G – have you ever felt **guilty** about your drinking?

E – have you ever had a drink first thing in the morning to steady the nerves (an **eye-opener**)?

Answering 'Yes' to two or more questions suggests a drinking problem. Once the problem has been identified, steps can be taken to rectify it.

- Cut down on alcohol intake – avoid pubs and wine bars; drink half-pints rather than pints; drink low-alcohol or alcohol-free drinks only; drink more slowly; start drinking later in the day; avoid other heavy drinkers; don't drink on an empty stomach; abstain for half a day or one day a week and gradually prolong this period.
- Join Alcoholics Anonymous or the local community alcohol team for support and guidance. The sister organization Al-Anon offers support and counselling to the families of alcoholics.
- If withdrawal problems occur – delirium tremens (DTs), tremor, sweats, weakness, abdominal cramps, nausea and vomiting – seek medical help.
- Many alcoholics tend to ignore their nutrition – start on general multivitamins and minerals.

Self-help for smokers

- Do you have a high tobacco dependence?
  smoking within 30 minutes of waking
  smoking more than 15 cigarettes daily
  craving cigarettes when unable to smoke
  previous unsuccessful attempts to stop smoking
  little confidence in ability to stop smoking
  never abstained for more than 1–2 days
  These more dependent smokers will have more difficulty in giving up.
- Most successful are people who stop at once – who decide on a 'quit date' and stick to it.
- Enlist the support of family and friends.
- Create no-smoking areas at home, work, etc.
- Remove all ashtrays from the immediate environment.
- Avoid situations and friends who are smokers.
- Take up exercise or a hobby to replace smoking.

- Keep a diary for a week before stopping. Detail every cigarette smoked and why.
- Take one day at a time.
- If stopping at once does not work, try cutting down slowly by smoking only a part of the cigarette; cutting cigarettes in half; smoking herbal cigarettes; buying smaller packets; stopping for one day a week and gradually increasing the smoke-free period.
- Collect the money otherwise spent on cigarettes in a glass jar. Keep the jar on a shelf within easy view.
- Some people carry an unopened packet with them so that they do not panic when they 'give in'. This works to relieve their anxiety – the person often finds they never open the packet.
- For withdrawal effects and craving use nicotine chewing gum or patches.
- Ring a helpline:

  Quit
  Tel. 0171 487 2858
  (Newsletters, advice on local resources)

  Quitline
  Tel. 0171 487 3000
  (Gives support and advice)

Self-help for prescription drug addiction

- Inform your doctor that you may be addicted to the drug – most commonly a tranquillizer.
- Stop other stimulants in the diet (e.g. tea, coffee, colas, cigarettes, alcohol) before attempting to cut down the drug.
- Do not stop abruptly. Come off the drug gradually. Halve the dose at first, then quarter it. Some people shave a little bit off the tablet with a razor blade each day to make withdrawal as painless as possible.
- Coming off tranquillizers can take months or years.

Conventional treatment

For alcohol addiction the first step is confirmation of the problem, followed by provision of medication to avoid DTs and fits (detoxification regimen) – usually a 1 week course of tranquillizers – as well as help with referral to Alcoholics Anonymous and support to the family. Doctors may also prescribe high-dose vitamin supplements.

Smokers are recommended to follow the general advice above. Eighty per cent will experience withdrawal symptoms – craving, irritability, anxiety, increased appetite, poor concentration, depression and restlessness. Private prescriptions for nicotine patches will save the patient from having to pay value-added tax (VAT) in the UK. Some general practitioners have carbon monoxide meters and can use these to monitor patients' smoking habits and whether patients are being truthful about their progress.

Complementary therapy

Acupressure
Press on points for 1–2 minutes to help with craving from nicotine withdrawal:
   Colon 4
   Liver 3
For point location see Chapter 2.

Acupuncture
Ear acupuncture can be very effective in helping nicotine craving and drug addiction. Acupuncture will also help to relieve anxiety and stress brought on by withdrawal.

Homoeopathy
- Alcohol withdrawal:
     aconite 6X half-hourly, maximum of 10 doses.
- Tranquilizers:
     anxiety, restlessness: arsenicum 6C every 15 minutes, maximum of 10 doses
     help with withdrawal: nux vomica 6X three times daily.

Hypnotherapy
Works well in some people to help stop smoking.

Naturopathy and nutrition
General advice and self-help is provided together with vitamin and mineral supplementation, especially vitamins A, B, C, D, K, folic acid, manganese, potassium, iron and cysteine (an amino acid found in nuts, seeds, dairy products and wholegrains). Oil of evening primrose may also be beneficial.

For withdrawal from drugs or alcohol the patient may need admission to a private clinic. Treatments include supplementation as well as detoxification by fasting, juicing, herbal and mineral baths, massage, relaxation methods and exercise.

Other therapies
Reflexology, meditation, Bach flower remedies and aromatherapy will all help in decreasing anxiety and help the patient come through the withdrawal period.

12

Complementary medicine and the medical profession

Medicolegal aspects

Who is liable if something goes wrong?

Overall the general practitioner retains clinical responsibility for the patient after referral to a non-medically qualified complementary therapist. There should be no problems if the referral is appropriate, i.e. if the doctor has taken a satisfactory medical history and examination and then referred.

For referral to a therapist the doctor should ensure:

- the therapist is sent a referral letter with all relevant clinical findings and investigations
- the therapist is registered with a recognized professional body which has a defined code of ethics, disciplinary and grievance procedures and a requirement for continous education and development
- the therapist has personal indemnity insurance (NHS therapists are usually covered by their employers)
- the therapist maintains regular communication with the GP to monitor patient therapy
- the patient is seen by the GP after an appropriate period to review the condition and discuss therapy.

A doctor can refuse to refer a patient to a complementary practitioner. If the patient then self-refers that is between the patient and the therapist. The doctor will not have contributed and will not be responsible for whatever transpires.

The doctor still retains the responsibility to see and treat a patient who has *already* seen a complementary therapist.

Doctors who are in doubt about their medicolegal standing should consult their medical defence organization.

The future

The British Medical Association in its 1993 report entitled *Complementary Medicine* made the following comments and recommendations:

- The present situation which allows anyone to practise freely, irrespective of training and experience, is unacceptable.
- If an unregulated practice poses a danger to patients it should require statutory regulation.
- Good and safe complementary therapies should be encouraged.
- A single regulating organization should represent each complementary therapy with a defined code of ethics, a system for communicating with GPs, disciplinary and grievance procedures and a requirement for continuous education and development.
- Recognized training should be established for each therapy with appropriate clinical and medical information.
- Research and development should be encouraged in all complementary fields.
- Postgraduate education (postgraduate education allowance (PGEA) approved) courses should be organized for doctors to illustrate the complementary techniques available and possible patient benefits.
- Doctors wishing to practise a complementary technique should undertake recognized training and only treat patients after registration with the professional body.

Glossary

Acute A condition arising suddenly, often with intense severity but quickly over.

Adhesions Tissues in the body stuck together, often as a result of infection or operation.

Analgesia Any kind of pain relief.

Anecdotal evidence 'Stories' that members of the medical profession and patients report – not subject to formal scientific scrutiny.

Angina Central chest pain or tightness when the blood supply to the heart becomes compromised, usually due to narrowed coronary arteries.

Case–control study Two groups are compared, one with the disease and one without. The two groups are matched as closely as possible for variables that may affect the possibility of getting the disease, such as age, sex, nationality, etc.

Cholesterol A constituent of cells. Essential for the manufacture of hormones and enzymes. Often described as a 'body fat'. Excess cholesterol can deposit in artery walls and cause narrowing which can lead to angina, heart attack and strokes.

Chronic Long-standing.

Cognitive therapy Therapy based on reasoning, perception and intuition.

Colitis Inflammation of the large intestine (colon). Can cause abdominal pain, and give rise to mucus and blood in the stool.

Colon The large intestine.

Congenital A condition that exists from birth.

Controlled trial Two groups are compared. The treated group receives the treatment (e.g. a drug) or intervention (e.g. a fat-free diet) and the control group does not.

Cortisol A hormone made by the adrenal glands which lie on top of the kidney. Helps the body deal with stress.

DNA Deoxyribonucleic acid. Contains the genetic material that codes each organism, making it different from the next. Exists in cells as chromosomes. Short areas of DNA in a chromosome that code for a particular characteristic are called genes.

Double-blind trial Of the groups being treated, neither researchers nor the patients know who is getting which treatment; some may be receiving placebo, some the real drug. This kind of trial prevents bias by researchers and patients.

Endorphins Morphine-like hormones released in the brain which help block the sensation of pain.

Fibre Carbohydrates occurring naturally in the diet that cannot be digested by humans. Fibre acts as a bulking agent and is useful in constipation and irritable bowel syndrome.

Gonadotrophins Hormones produced by the pituitary gland in the brain that stimulate the testicles and ovaries to produce sperm, eggs and sex hormones.

Healing crisis A recurrence of symptoms caused by the elimination of toxins from the body. Usually occurs after the first session of a complementary therapy.

Homoeostasis The maintenance of a constant internal environment by self-regulation.

Hyperlipidaemia Abnormally high levels of lipids (fats) and cholesterol in the blood.

Inflammation The response of tissues to injury. Symptoms include redness, warmth, pain and swelling. Denoted by the ending '-itis', e.g. cellulitis, appendicitis.

In-vitro study Research carried out in a laboratory without the use of a living organism.

In-vivo study Research carried out on a living organism.

Iris The coloured portion of the eye. Contraction and expansion of its muscles cause the pupil to change size and control the amount of light entering the eye.

Ischaemia Lack of oxygen to the muscles, as in ischaemic heart disease: less blood reaches the heart muscle and angina ensues.

Leucocyte Any kind of white blood cell.

Meta-analysis A study combining the results of many smaller studies in the hope of establishing a conclusive result.

Perineum That part of the muscular floor of the pelvis that lies between the top of the thighs.

Phagocytosis The destruction of bacteria, viruses or other foreign bodies by surrounding, engulfing and digesting – like an amoeba.

Placebo A pharmacologically inactive substance used in research. Often made to look like the actual drug under study. Patients (and often researchers) are unaware if they are taking the true drug or the placebo.

Randomized trial Subjects are assigned to different groups randomly without bias.

Statistically significant Unlikely to be due to chance.

Sciatica Pain and tingling down the leg – over the buttock, down the leg and to the outer edge of the foot to the little toe. Caused by pressure on the sciatic nerve in the lower back.

Index

248   Index